Professional Ethics:
A Guide for Rehabilitation Professionals

Professional Ethics:
A Guide for Rehabilitation Professionals

Ron Scott, JD, PT, OCS

Associate Professor
Physical Therapy Department, School of Allied Health Sciences
University of Texas Health Science Center
San Antonio, Texas

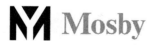 Mosby

St. Louis Baltimore Boston Carlsbad Chicago Minneapolis New York Philadelphia Portland
London Milan Sydney Tokyo Toronto

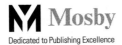

Mosby

Dedicated to Publishing Excellence

A Times Mirror Company

Publisher: John Schrefer
Executive Editor: Martha Sasser
Developmental Editor: Christie Hart
Project Manager: Gayle Morris
Manufacturing Manager: Karen Lewis
Cover Designer: Dave Zielinski

Printed in the United States of America
Design, production, and composition: GraphCom Corporation
Printing and binding: RR Donnelley

Mosby, Inc.
11830 Westline Industrial Drive
St. Louis, MO 63146

International Standard Book Number 0-8151-2525-9

98 99 00 01 02 / 9 8 7 6 5 4 3 2 1

This book is dedicated to the late and incomparable
Selena Quintanilla Perez, a consummate professional,
whose adherence to the highest standards of
professional ethics tragically cost the entertainer her
life at the advent of superstardom. Thank you for your
immeasurable contributions and for being an
inspiration to, and role model for, people of all ages,
races and ethnicity, and social status. You will always
be among us.

Foreword

When bioethics was born nearly 30 years ago, its pioneers observed that technology often posed difficult moral questions, even as it created new and powerful ways of treating or preventing illness. That observation is as true today as it was 3 decades ago. Two additional changes, however, have complicated matters even farther. First, there have been dramatic, some would say revolutionary, changes in the way health care is organized and financed. Pressures to keep down costs lead to demands to prove the value of every intervention, to maximize efficiency, and, in many cases, to do less rather than more. The second change is the belated recognition that physicians are not the only health care professionals. Together, those changes make a book such as this a necessity.

Rehabilitation professionals, like other health care professionals, work in an increasingly complex environment. What seemed obvious and easy a decade ago now may seem obscure and difficult. What are my ethical duties? What are my legal responsibilities? Called to a healing art, rehabilitation professionals have ethical and legal loyalties to their patients. Those loyalties may be difficult at times to reconcile with organizational priorities, financial pressures, and personal needs or wants. Rehabilitation professionals, as with other health professionals, face complex and vexing problems. At times the problem may be mostly a matter of law, with little ethical content. Most of the time, however, ethical and legal implications will be closely intertwined. *Professional Ethics: A Guide for Rehabilitation Professionals* recognizes this and discusses both ethics and law, the deep connections between the two but also their differences. The book is a praiseworthy effort to provide wisdom and guidance at a time when both are sorely needed.

Thomas H. Murray, PhD
Professor and Director
Center for Biomedical Ethics
Case Western Reserve University

About the Author

Ron Scott is an associate professor in the Department of Physical Therapy, School of Allied Health Sciences, University of Texas Health Science Center at San Antonio. Ron teaches Professional Ethics, Patient Care I, Management and Administration, and Differential Diagnosis.

Ron is also an adjunct professor in the Master of Arts in Health Services Management program at Webster University, where he teaches Human Resource Management and Law and Health Services courses. He also has a consulting law and risk management practice.

Ron retired from the army in 1994, where he was a Judge Advocate General (JAG) Corps officer and physical therapist–clinician and manager. He has been married since 1973 to Maria Josefa ("Pepi") Barba Garces. They have two sons, Ron, Jr., an English major at the University of North Texas, and Paul, a freshman at Southwest Texas State University.

Ron is past chair of the American Physical Therapy Association's Judicial Committee; a legal faculty member of APTA's risk management program; editor, Section on Geriatrics, *Issues on Aging;* and a member of the Editorial Advisory Board for *PT: The Magazine of Physical Therapy.* He has written over 70 articles on orthopedics, quality and risk management, human resources management, and law and ethics. This is Ron's fourth book. His other books are *Promoting Legal Awareness in Physical and Occupational Therapy* (Mosby, 1997), *Legal Aspects of Documenting Patient Care* (Aspen, 1994), and *Health Care Malpractice: A Primer on Legal Issues* (Slack, 1990).

In his spare time, Ron likes to travel, play guitar, collect Beatles paraphernalia, and write comedy and fiction works.

Preface

This book addresses issues in health professional ethics. Professional ethics refers to official conduct of members of a profession, which is normally governed by a code of ethical conduct promulgated by a professional association.

Although the book is particularly targeted toward rehabilitation professionals—physical and occupational therapists and assistants, prosthetists and orthotists and assistants, rehabilitation nurses, respiratory therapists, and speech-language pathologists and audiologists, the principles explored are acutely relevant for other professionals involved in patient care, including, but not limited to, physicians, physician assistants, nurses in practice settings other than physical rehabilitation, clinical laboratory professionals, dentists and dental hygenists and assistants, chiropractors, emergency medical technicians, clinical managers, health care administrators, and health law attorneys. The principles and issues discussed in this book will also be of interest to the public-at-large, particularly those of us who are or may become patients within the health care system at some point in our lives (or are close to someone who is, or will, become a patient).

Health care professionals are special-status professionals. There are no other endeavors on earth in which clients—in their most vulnerable physical, mental, emotional, and spiritual states—place their lives in the hands of others for therapeutic intervention. Caring for patients is a sacred calling. Health professionals at all levels are fiduciaries, who owe their highest duty to patients under their care.

New health care delivery paradigms, including managed care, have created serious conflicts involving duties owed by health care professionals to patients, employing entities, and themselves. The law and principles of professional ethics have not changed substantially (nor should they) to accommodate the business of managed care.

Careful adherence by health professionals to the ethical principles that govern official conduct will enable the health care delivery system to thrive and continue to evolve into a better system, for patients and their significant others, for providers and support professionals, for society, and for civilization.

Acknowledgments

I wish to thank my wife, Maria Josefa (Pepi) Scott Barba-Garces, for her encouragement, patience, and love during the development of this manuscript and throughout all of my professional endeavors.

I also wish to thank Dr. William Moore, Jr., Professor, The University of Texas at Austin, in whose Ethics and Values graduate class I was constantly challenged and inspired.

Finally, I would like to thank those involved at Mosby for their efforts: Martha Sasser, Kellie White, Leah Hiner, Christie Hart, and Dana Peick.

Table of Contents

Table of Contents

Professional Ethics:
A Guide for Rehabilitation Professionals

Introduction

This chapter defines and describes morals, ethics, and law; it describes the four foundational biomedical ethical principles of beneficence, nonmaleficence, justice, and autonomy; it offers a systems approach to health care professional ethical decision making. The five bases of legal duty are also explored, including constitutional, statutory authority, and judicial case law; regulatory authority; and secondary legal sources (including professional practice standards and codes of ethics, among others). This chapter also addresses the modern "blending" of legal and professional ethical obligations, under which a substantive violation of law by a health care provider more often than not also constitutes a violation of professional ethics.

•

Bases for Ethical Conduct

Morals

Morals refers to beliefs, principles, and values about what is right and what is wrong, which are personal to each and every individual. A person's moral beliefs are often—but not always—grounded in religion. Morals may also be grounded in secular philosophic theories about right and wrong. One can be a moral person without being a religious person.

Morals, like ethics, are culture-based and culture-driven, as well as time-dependent. There are only a few universal (or near-universal) morals, including the prohibitions against murder, rape, and incest, and the moral duty to treat others as you would like to be treated.

No one is or should feel compelled to abide by another person's morality, although individuals are clearly obliged to comply with organized ethical and legal mandates. Morals are exclusively *intra*personal in nature. One is acting with moral virtue, or character, when he or she strives to "do the right thing."

Ethics

Ethics refers to how individuals conduct themselves in their personal and professional endeavors. The word *ethics* derives from the Greek words *ethikos*, which means character, and *ethos*, which means custom. Ethical rules of conduct are firmly grounded in moral theory.

People face problems, issues, and dilemmas with ethical dimensions, which necessitate action (or nonaction) every day. **Problems** involve questions of conduct, which are relatively straightforward, temporary in nature, and readily resolvable. **Issues** involve points of debate or controversy having strong sentiments on two (or more) sides, which are normally resolved through compromise by finding a "middle ground." **Dilemmas** entail situations wherein decision makers are faced with two (or more) equally favorable or unfavorable alternative options for possible implementation. Examples of problems, issues, and dilemmas include the following:

- Clinical practice *problems* faced by a physical therapist involving whether to carry out or seek modification of a physician treatment order for a patient that calls for less-than-optimal therapeutic intervention by the therapist
- *Issues* of whether to pursue a legal remedy for possible encroachment on professional practice by members of a related health professional discipline
- *Dilemmas* of deciding whether to accept or challenge a physician's invocation and application of therapeutic privilege (an exception to the normal requirement for patient informed consent to treatment, discussed in detail in Chapters 3 and 10) involving a particular patient's care

No one is or should feel compelled to abide by another person's morality... Morals are exclusively intrapersonal in nature. One is acting with moral virtue, or character, when he or she strives to "do the right thing."

2

There are three fundamental elements to any ethical problem, issue, or dilemma. There is an agent, or *actor,* who is faced with a problem, issue, or dilemma. The actor must engage in some sort of *conduct* involving action or nonaction. Further, there is an *effect,* or consequence, associated with the actor's conduct related to the problem, issue, or dilemma.

Ethical theorists have analyzed these fundamental elements of actor, conduct, and effect to develop and refine their classical ethical theories. (A theory involves a set of assumptions used by theorists to explain or predict phenomena. A theory cannot be proved; it can only be disproved.) Box 1-1 lists and briefly describes the principal classical ethical theories.

Box 1-1. Classical Ethical Theories

Teleological (consequentialism [*telos,* Greek for *end* or *goal*]) **ethics.** The moral quality of conduct is assessed by focusing on its effects or consequences. *Utilitarianism*—the tailoring of one's conduct so as to affect the greatest social good with a minimum of adverse consequences—is one expression of consequentialism. Whether an actor affects the greatest social utility by carefully obeying established legal and ethical rules of conduct *(rule utilitarianism)* or by merely conducting himself or herself subjectively in such a way as to affect the greatest good, irrespective of the *rules (act utilitarianism),* is a matter of opinion.

Deontological (*deon,* Greek for *duty*) **ethics.** The nature of conduct is prospectively assessed, using established universal standards for behavior, including religious commandments and edicts, professional ethics codes, and rules of civil and criminal law. Under a deontological ethics approach, an actor fulfills his or her duty by following the *rules,* without focusing on the consequences of conduct.

Deonutility ethics.[1] This approach to ethics combines the ethical theories of teleology (consequentialism) and deontology, under which good principles and guidance are believed to bring good results.

Virtue ethics. This approach focuses on actors and their character and judgment and relations with other people, rather than specifically on rules or consequences of conduct.

Law

Everyone in society (with the possible exception of persons having diplomatic immunity) has an affirmative duty to comply with the administrative, civil, and criminal laws in effect in the jurisdiction. It is often said that "ignorance of the law is no excuse" for noncompliance. Whereas real problems exist in society regarding the

3

selective enforcement of laws, every person—from the homeless pauper to the President of the United States—is bound by the laws of the land.

Even diplomats are not always assured immunity from answering for their conduct under the law. Consider the case of Georgy Makharadze, a Georgian diplomat who was involved in a traffic accident in Washington, D.C., in December, 1996. Largely because of political pressure from the United States State Department, President Eduard Shevardnadze waived diplomatic immunity for Makharadze in February, 1997, freeing the way for his possible prosecution for vehicular homicide in the case.[2]

Sources of law and legal obligation. There are four primary sources of law and legal obligation in society: constitutional law authority, statutory law authority, case law authority, and administrative or regulatory authority. There are also many potential secondary sources of legal authority and obligation. A depiction of the hierarchy of sources of law and legal authority appears in Figure 1-1.

Constitutional law. The preeminent source of legal authority is the federal Constitution, known as the "supreme law of the land." All other laws, rules, and regulations—including international treaties—are subordinate in authority to the express provisions of the Constitution and to the interpretations of federal constitution-

It is often said that "ignorance of the law is no excuse" for noncompliance.

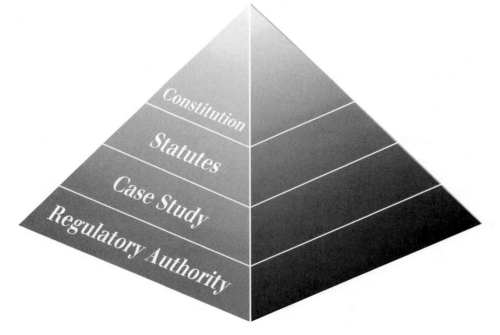

Figure 1-1. Sources of law and legal authority.

al law rendered by the courts. Although there exists a historical controversy concerning which federal branch has ultimate constitutional interpretive authority, the United States Supreme Court is generally recognized as the final arbiter in interpreting and enforcing the Constitution.

Many legal cases interpreting the Constitution throughout the history of the United States have impacted health care delivery, including cases concerning the nature and scope of *due process* of law (rules of fundamental fairness, including notice of hearing and the right to be heard concerning governmental actions affecting the liberty, property, and lives of private citizens) and cases concerning the fundamental right of individual privacy. *Griswold v. Connecticut,*[3] the 1965 case in which the United States Supreme Court first ruled that there was a fundamental privacy right, centered on the right of conjugate adult partners to legally purchase pharmaceutical contraceptives for birth control. The creation of the fundamental right of individual privacy is the first and only instance in which the United States Supreme Court found an implied (versus express) federal constitutional right.

Virtually all of the express written provisions concerning individual rights and liberties are contained not in the main body but in the amendments to the federal Constitution. Individual rights and liberties were not addressed by the founding fathers during the original Constitutional Convention in 1787 but were added as amendments to the Constitution in 1791 and modeled substantially after the Virginia Bill of Rights. The first ten Constitutional amendments—collectively known as the Bill of Rights— were originally intended to protect private citizens and the states from over-regulation by the federal government. The Bill of Rights is reprinted in Box 1-2.

Box 1-2. Bill of Rights

Amendment I: Congress shall make no law respecting an establishment of religion, or prohibiting the free exercise thereof; or abridging the freedom of speech, or of the press; or the right of the people peaceably to assemble, and to petition the Government for a redress of grievances.

Amendment II: A well regulated Militia, being necessary to the security of a free State, the right of the people to keep and bear Arms, shall not be infringed.

Amendment III: No quartering of soldiers in private homes during peacetime. (Obsolete, but still in force.)

Amendment IV: The right of the people to be secure in their persons, houses, papers, and effects, against unreasonable searches and seizures, shall not be violated, and no Warrants shall issue, but upon probable cause, supported by Oath or affirmation and particularly describing the place to be searched, and the persons or things to be seized.

Box 1-2. Bill of Rights—cont'd

Amendment V: No person shall be held to answer for a capital, or otherwise infamous crime, unless on a presentment or indictment of a Grand Jury, except in cases arising in the land or naval forces, or in the Militia, when in actual service in time of War or public danger; nor shall any person be subject for the same offense to be twice put in jeopardy of life or limb; nor shall be compelled in any criminal case to be a witness against himself, not be deprived of life, liberty, or property, without due process of law; nor shall private property be taken for public use, without just compensation.

Amendment VI: In all criminal prosecutions, the accused shall enjoy the right to a speedy and public trial, by an impartial jury of the State and district wherein the crime shall have been committed, which district shall have been previously ascertained by law, and to be informed of the nature and cause of the accusation; to be confronted with the witnesses against him; to have compulsory process for obtaining witnesses in his favor, and to have the Assistance of Counsel for his defense.

Amendment VII: In Suits at common law, where the value in controversy shall exceed twenty dollars, the right of trial by jury shall be preserved, and no fact tried by jury, shall be otherwise reexamined in any Court of the United States, than according to the rules of the common law.

Amendment VIII: Excessive bail shall not be required, nor excessive fines imposed, nor cruel and unusual punishments inflicted.

Amendment IX: The enumeration in the Constitution, of certain rights, shall not be construed to deny or disparage others retained by the people.

Amendment X: The powers not delegated to the United States by the Constitution, nor prohibited by it to the States, are reserved to the States respectively, or to the people.

State constitutional law, although subordinate to federal constitutional law, is supreme to conflicting state statutory and regulatory law. States may grant their citizens and residents greater rights than are granted under the federal Constitution, but they cannot derogate from the basic federal rights, privileges, and immunities granted to citizens and residents by the federal Constitution.

Statutory law. The second primary source of legal authority is statutory law. Congress and the state legislatures enact statutes within their spheres of legal authority. Federal statutes, published in the United States Code (USC), are divided by general subjects into "titles." Examples of some of the important federal statutes affecting health care delivery include the Americans with Disabilities Act of 1990, the Civil Rights Acts of 1964 and 1991, the Family and Medical Leave Act of 1993, the Patient Self-Determination Act of 1990, the Privacy Act of 1974, and the Rehabilitation

Act of 1973. State statutes enacted by state legislative bodies are controlling laws in areas where the states, and not the federal government, have jurisdiction (control). Examples of state statutes include those creating and regulating the licensure of health professionals and insurance statutes.

Case law. The third primary source of legal authority is judge-made case law, or common law. The common law creates legal authority in all areas wherein constitutions and legislation have not created legal precedent. Many common law legal precedents are still based on early English common law. Most American civil legal authority derives from common law, including laws related to health care legal and ethical issues, business relationships among health professionals and organizations, and others.

Although the common law is traditionally viewed as being relatively more flexible and quick to adapt to societal changes than other sources of legal authority, the common law is still relatively stable. The concept called *stare decisis,* meaning "the decision stands," requires all subordinate courts in a jurisdiction (i.e., in a particular state or a federal circuit) to abide by prior decisions on a point of law rendered by a higher-level court within the jurisdiction. Permanent changes in the status quo, then, occur only when the highest courts in a jurisdiction modify or overturn existing precedential case law authority.

Administrative law. The final primary source of legal authority is administrative or regulatory agencies at the local, state, and federal levels. Regulatory agencies exercise authority delegated to them by the legislative and executive branches of government. They are empowered to exercise legislative (rule making), executive (management), and judicial (enforcement) roles. In their legislative role, regulatory agencies promulgate administrative rules and regulations that supplement statutes and executive orders. At the federal level, such rules and regulations are normally previewed for public review and comment in the *Federal Register* and are eventually published in final form in the *Code of Federal Regulations* (CFR).

Once in final form, administrative rules and regulations exert significant influence over business conduct. It is widely accepted as fact that health care professionals in all practice, research, and educational settings have greater everyday interface with regulatory agencies than with all other legal entities combined.

Examples of federal administrative agencies having broad authority over health care business affairs include the Centers for Disease Control (CDC), the Equal Employment Opportunity Commission (EEOC), the Health Care Financing Administration (HCFA), the Occupational Safety and Health Administration (OSHA), the National Labor Relations Board (NLRB), and the Social Security Administration (SSA). Examples of state administrative agencies affecting health care professionals and delivery of health care services include agencies administering health professional licensure, state insurance commissions, and workers' compensation authorities.

7

Secondary legal authorities. Additional (secondary) sources of law, on which legislative, executive, judicial, and administrative governmental decision makers may rely as "authorities," include, among others, professional association practice and ethics standards; professional and institutional clinical practice protocols and guidelines; and accreditation standards promulgated by private organizations such as the Joint Commission on Accreditation of Healthcare Organizations (JCAHO), the Commission on Accreditation of Rehabilitation Facilities (CARF), and the National Committee on Quality Assurance (NCQA).

Health Professional, Business, and Organizational Ethics Defined and Distinguished

Every individual comports his or her official conduct with personal or group ethical standards. These standards of conduct may differ markedly, depending on the nature of the person's occupation, profession, or position.

Business ethics addresses standards of conduct for business people and organizations in general. In sociocapitalist societies, like the United States, Canada, Mexico, Japan, the European community of nations, and others, the coprimary missions of private business organizations are: (1) to generate monetary profits, and (2) to meet express and implied social responsibilities. Social responsibility includes acts in the public interest, from affirmative action employment practices to civic charity to support for the arts to volunteerism, among a myriad of other activities.

Health professional ethical standards differ from general business ethical standards in several ways. Most health care entities are organized as not-for-profit businesses and therefore strive to generate net income (revenue over expenses)[4] but not profits. Additionally, health care professionals treat patients who are injured or suffer from disease and are in pain and who therefore are more vulnerable to exploitation than the overwhelming majority of ordinary business clients. Health professionals are required by law and ethical standards to maintain diagnostic, historical, and treatment-related patient information in strict confidence. The delivery of health care to patients is often emergent, and the consequences of bad decisions are potentially dire. For all these reasons and more, the legal and ethical standards of conduct for health care professionals are intentionally set extremely high—higher than for most other business pursuits.

Managed care has created a number of ethical dilemmas for health professionals and organizations who are *fiduciaries* for their patients, meaning that they are trustees, who must place the interests of their patients above their own. From financial conflicts of interest involving provider variable or incentive pay for limiting patient care costs to "gag clauses," which inhibit free provider-patient communications, managed care has given rise to a number of significant ethical problems, issues,

Health care professionals treat patients who are injured or suffer from disease and are in pain and who therefore are more vulnerable to exploitation than the overwhelming majority of ordinary business clients. The delivery of health care to patients is often emergent, and the consequences of bad decisions are potentially dire.

and dilemmas. These managed care ethical concerns are addressed in appropriate chapters throughout this text.

What are the attributes of a *profession?* A profession has the following characteristics[5,6]:

- **Defined body of accrued knowledge or expertise.** (The *classic* [original] *professions*—law, medicine, and the clergy—were described as having unique domains of knowledge and expertise, so that no one else could carry out the professional roles of their members. Modernly, there are many, many more than three *professions.*)

- **Autonomy,** or self-governance, including the establishment and enforcement of a *code of ethics* and quality standards for the professional product or service (e.g., *standards of practice* for the health professions)

- **Formal education** of its members

- **Research activities** designed to validate and refine professional practice

- Existence of one or more **professional societies** or **organizations** for the development of the profession and its members

- **Recognition of advanced member competency** through certification or other processes

Two other terms related to health care professional ethics warrant definition. **Bioethics** is a term used to define the identification, analysis, and resolution of ethical problems, issues, and dilemmas associated with the biological sciences, especially medicine and health care practice and research.[7] **Clinical ethics** relates specifically to ethical problems, issues, and dilemmas associated with clinical patient care activities.[8,9]

Modern Blending of Law and Professional Ethics

Modernly, law and ethics have been largely blended into common standards of professional conduct. Often, professional conduct that constitutes a breach of ethics also constitutes a violation of law, and visa versa. Figure 1-2 illustrates the nature of the modern blending of legal and professional ethical responsibilities.

Part of the rationale for the modern blending of law and health professional ethics is that society has become highly legalistic in recent times. United States citizens and residents claim against and sue one another more than anywhere else in the world. For example, in 1992 there were 19,707,374 new civil lawsuits filed nationwide.[10] Coupled with a presumed equal number of existing civil lawsuits in the system, as many as one in seven Americans may be embroiled in civil litigation at any given time.

Another reason for the mixed nature of law and health professional ethics is the fact that patients and other consumers of health care services and exper-

A profession has an autonomous body of accrued knowledge; it enforces a code of ethics and offers standards of practice; it provides education for its members and is involved in research activities; it promotes organizations for the development of its members; and it recognizes advanced competency.

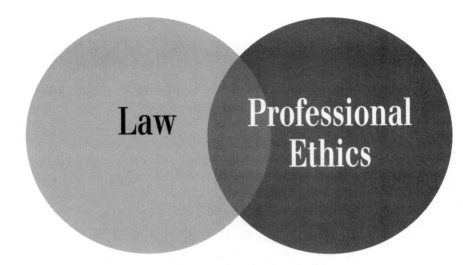

Figure 1-2. Modern blending of law and professional ethics.

tise have become more sophisticated in recent times. Patients are more aware of their rights as consumers and are more disposed to assert those rights, including the use of the legal system.

There are at least four potential venues for processing alleged violations of law and professional ethics by health care professionals. Consider the following hypothetical example:

> A physical therapist in private practice is charged by a patient with sexual misconduct. The specific allegation involves alleged fondling of the patient's breasts by the therapist during a treatment session. The patient was properly referred to the therapist by an orthopedic surgeon for postoperative rotator cuff repair rehabilitation.

In which forums might disciplinary action ensue? The patient may pursue civil (private) and criminal legal actions against the physical therapist. Although the patient can initiate a civil lawsuit for health care malpractice (based on intentional misconduct), the filing of a criminal case is normally discretionary with the local state prosecutor after the filing of the patient's criminal complaint.

The sanctions in a civil malpractice trial after a finding of liability by a preponderance, or greater weight, of evidence include compensatory money damages that are designed to make the injured plaintiff-patient whole (including medical expenses, lost earnings, and pain and suffering) and punitive damages (intended to punish the offender and dissuade others from following in his or her footsteps). The sanctions in a criminal case, after a finding of guilt beyond a reasonable doubt, include incarceration or the threat of incarceration (e.g., probation or a suspended sentence of imprisonment) and a monetary fine, which is the criminal court analog to civil punitive money damages.

The physical therapist may also face adverse administrative action by his or her state licensure board. If culpability is established before the licensure board by a preponderance of evidence, the sanction may include licensure suspension or revocation.

Finally, the therapist may face action by his or her professional association for a violation of the applicable code of professional ethics. Upon a finding of culpability by a preponderance of evidence, sanctions—along a continuum of possible sanctions—may include probation (with or without conditions), suspension, or revocation of membership in the professional association.

Legal and Ethical Health Care Four-Quadrant Clinical Practice Grid

The legal and ethical health care four-quadrant clinical practice grid (Figure 1-3) illustrates acceptable and unacceptable health care clinical practice, based on compliance with or violation of legal and ethical practice rules and standards. The same model can also be applied to health care professionals in academia and research settings.

It is relatively easy to delineate clinical practice that clearly meets or violates legal and ethical rules and standards. For example, a Certified Prosthetist-Orthotist (CPO) who practices in compliance with applicable state and federal laws and the Canons of Ethical Conduct of the American Board for Certification (ABC) is practicing in a manner that meets legal and ethical requirements. If the same provider is charged with and admits to sexual misconduct with a patient, then he or she has complied with neither legal nor ethical standards. These modes of practice can be labeled +L/+E and −L/−E, respectively.

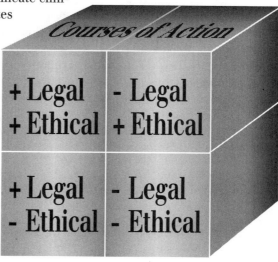

Figure 1-3. Legal and ethical health care four-quadrant clinical practice grid.

11

Professional conduct may be a violation of ethical standards but not a violation of the law or +L/−E practice. Consider the following example:

> An employment contract between a physician and a managed care organization contains a provision that prohibits the physician from discussing with patients treatment options that are not offered by the managed care organization. (Such a contractual provision is commonly referred to as a "gag clause," which is discussed in greater detail in Chapter 3.) Even if compliance with the "gag clause" by the physician might be upheld by a court as a legally acceptable course of action, such conduct would still constitute an actionable breach of professional ethics. Under applicable ethical standards governing patient informed consent to treatment, a competent patient must be informed by a physician of *all* reasonable alternatives to a proposed intervention, irrespective of whether a managed care organization elects to offer them as a matter of its business judgment. The provider in this case might face adverse administrative or American Medical Association (AMA) action for a breach of professional ethics, in spite of the legality of the contract.

The most difficult mode of clinical practice to describe involves official conduct by a clinician that meets professional ethics standards but violates legal requirements, the −L/+E mode of practice. Some legal and ethics scholars might argue that a breach of professional ethics also occurs any time a health professional's conduct violates the law. However, consider the example of a physical therapist in independent practice (PTIP) who treats an indigent Medicare patient in an outpatient setting. Ignorant of any possible regulatory prohibition against doing so, the physical therapist waives the patient's Medicare Part B copayment for 20 percent of the charges but submits a bill to Medicare for its 80 percent contribution to the patient's bill. The physical therapist is clearly complying with Principle 8, Section 8.1 of the American Physical Therapy Association's (APTA) Guide for Professional Conduct,[11] which reads:

> *8.1 Pro Bono Service.* Physical therapists should render pro bono publico (reduced or no fee) services to patients lacking the ability to pay for services, as each physical therapist's practice permits.

However, the physical therapist might be in violation of federal administrative rules promulgated by the Health Care Financing Administration (HCFA), which generally prohibit the waiver of Part B Medicare patient copayments.

Health care professionals should consider their professional conduct in light of the four-quadrant grid and strive always to be clearly in compliance with both legal and ethical mandates.

"Situational" Ethics

A foundational ethics question is the question of whether ethical rules and standards of conduct apply all of the time or are flexible enough to be disregarded in special situations. Situational ethics involves selective noncompliance with ethics rules and standards for special circumstances.

> **Situational ethics: Selective noncompliance by a professional with ethics rules and standards.**

There are two general circumstances that may cause a health care professional to practice situational ethics. First, a health care provider may elect not to comply with an ethical directive out of a sense of caring for a patient, colleague, or some other person. According to Fletcher,[12] this type of situational ethics occurs because of the health care professional's *agape* concern for the welfare of a patient (*agape,* Greek for *love for others*). Consider the following hypothetical example:

> O, an occupational therapist employed by ABC Medical Center is treating G, a 53-year-old female patient, who is diagnosed with mild right lower limb hemiplegia incident to a left cerebrovascular accident. G is ambulatory with a standard cane and is involved in group therapy to improve performance of activities of daily living (ADLs) in the kitchen environment. O learned in a rehabilitation team conference that G also is diagnosed with a malignant astrocytoma of the cerebellum. G's physiatrist, P, imposed a gag order, based on therapeutic privilege (discussed in detail in Chapter 3), on members of the rehabilitation team—including O—that requires them to refrain from discussing G's diagnosis or prognosis with her at this time. During the group therapy session, G finds herself alone with O for a moment and remarks that she sometimes feels dizzy. G asks, "I don't have a brain tumor or anything like that, do I?" O answers, "Of course not! Don't worry about such a thing!"

Has O violated professional ethics rules or standards? Principle 5C of the Occupational Therapy Code of Ethics[13] states that:

> Occupational therapy personnel shall refrain from using or participating in the use of any form of communication that contains false, fraudulent, deceptive, or unfair statements or claims.

13

Does compliance with the physiatrist's invocation of therapeutic privilege constitute an exception to Principle 5C of the Occupational Therapy Code of Ethics? That question must be answered, if it arises, by members of the American Occupational Therapy Association's (AOTA) Commission on Standards and Ethics. Assume for sake of argument that the occupational therapist's conduct is deemed by the Commission on Standards and Ethics not to be violative of the Occupational Therapy Code of Ethics. Nevertheless, the conduct of the occupational therapist may still violate his or her own personal ethical standards. If, for instance, the occupational therapist believes, like deontologist Immanuel Kant,[14] that truthfulness is a universally applicable *categorical imperative,* then the therapist has acted unethically by lying, even though the lie was occasioned by the physiatrist's order based on therapeutic privilege.

Situational ethics may also apply when a health care professional breaches professional ethics for reasons other than patient welfare, including out of malice or self-interest. Consider again the earlier example (under "Legal and Ethical Practice Grid") involving a physician's managed care employment gag clause provision, which disallowed the physician from discussing with patients care options not offered by the patients' health insurance plans. Compliance with the gag clause—in violation of AMA guidance—involves placing the physician's employment interests above patient welfare and constitutes *ethical relativism,* or *sliding scale* ethics.

Is it possible to practice situational ethics and still be ethical? That question must be individually answered by each professional. Although every health care professional succumbs to human frailty and breaches professional ethics at some point(s) during his or her career, it may be merely rationalization to create *situations* under which the breach of professional ethics is routinely acceptable.

Biomedical Ethical Principles

Health care professionals are guided by four foundational biomedical ethical principles in caring for patients (or conducting clinical research or educating professional students to care for patients). These four principles are beneficence, nonmaleficence, justice, and autonomy.[15] Each principle is discussed in turn and again in Chapter 3, because each principle relates to patient and research-subject informed consent issues.

Beneficence. Acting out of **beneficence** for a patient involves official conduct carried out in the patient's "best interests" by a health care provider. Beneficence is the manifestation of the health care professional's fiduciary duty owed to his or her patients. The Hippocratic Oath is reflective of the imperative that physicians, nurses, and allied health professionals are bound to act in patients' best interests in clinical health care delivery. It reads:

I swear...that I will fulfill according to my ability and judgment this oath and this covenant:

To hold him who has taught me this art as equal to my parents and to live my life in partnership with him, and if he is in need of money, to give him a share of mine, and to regard his offspring as equal to my brothers... and to teach them this art—if they desire to learn it—without fee and covenant....

I will apply dietetic measures for the benefit of the sick according to my ability and judgment; I will keep them from harm and injustice.

I will neither give a deadly drug to anybody if asked for it, nor will I make a suggestion to this effect. Similarly I will not give to a woman an abortive remedy. In purity and holiness I will guard my life and my art.

I will not use the knife, not even on sufferers from stone, but will withdraw in favor of such men as are engaged in this work.

Whatever houses I may visit, *I will come for the benefit of the sick* [emphasis added], remaining free of all intentional injustice, of all mischief and in particular of sexual relations with both female and male persons, be they free or slaves.

What I may see or hear in the course of the treatment or even outside of the treatment in regard to the life of men, which on no account one must spread abroad, I will keep to myself holding such things shameful to be spoken about.

If I fulfill this oath and do not violate it, may it be granted to me to enjoy life and art, being honored with fame among all men for all time to come; if I transgress it and swear falsely, may the opposite of all this be my lot.

Medical ethics, and health care ethics generally, have undergone a tremendous metamorphosis over time from an early deontological focus on strict compliance by physicians with the provisions of law and ethics, like the Hippocratic Oath, to a modern day period of analytical principlism,[16] under which health care professionals carefully consider the effects of their professional conduct before acting. This modern attitude is reflected, in part, in the Patient-Physician Covenant[17] (Box 1-3).

Box 1-3. Patient-Physician Covenant

Medicine is, at its center, a moral enterprise grounded in a covenant of trust. This covenant obliges physicians to be competent and to use their competence in the patient's best interests. Physicians, therefore, are both intellectually and morally obliged to act as advocates for the sick wherever their welfare is threatened and for their health at all times.

Today, this covenant of trust is significantly threatened. From within, there is growing legitimation of the physician's materialistic self-interest; from without, for-profit forces press the doctor into the role of commercial agent to enhance

---

Box 1-3. Patient-Physician Covenant—cont'd

the profitability of health care organizations. Such distortions of the doctor's responsibility degrade the doctor/patient relationship which is the central element and structure of clinical care. To capitulate to these alterations of the trust relationship is to significantly alter the doctor's role as healer, carer, helper and advocate for the sick, and for the health of all.

By its traditions and very nature, medicine is a special kind of human activity—one which cannot be pursued effectively without the virtues of humility, honesty, intellectual integrity, compassion and effacement of excessive self-interest. These traits mark doctors as members of a moral community dedicated to something other than its own self-interest.

Our first obligation must be to serve the good of those persons who seek our help and trust us to provide it. Physicians, as physicians, are not and must never be commercial entrepreneurs, gateclosers, or agents of fiscal policy that runs counter to our trust. Any defection from primacy of the patient's well-being places the patient at risk by treatment which may compromise quality of or access to medical care.

We believe the medical profession must reaffirm the primacy of its obligation to the patient through national, state, and local professional societies, our academic, research and hospital organizations, and especially through personal behavior. As advocates for the promotion of health and support of the sick we are called upon to discuss, defend and promulgate medical care by every ethical means available. Only by caring and advocating for the patient can the integrity of our profession be affirmed. Thus we honor our covenant of trust with patients.*

Nonmaleficence. **Nonmaleficence** means to *do no harm.* Health care interventions carried out on patients' behalf, however, may cause them to suffer pain or other injury. The ethical principle of nonmaleficence requires that the health care provider not *intentionally* cause harm or injury to patients under his or her care. Dr. Jack Kevorkian would assert that he does not violate the fundamental biomedical ethical principle of nonmaleficence in assisting his clients to die because his sole purpose in intervening is to alleviate the patients' suffering.

---

*This Covenant was produced by a group of American physicians, including Dr. David Rogers (deceased), who was former Dean of Medicine at Johns Hopkins and former President of the Robert Wood Johnson Foundation, and also including Dr. Christine Cassel, who is now Professor of Medicine at the University of Chicago. Dr. Edmund Pelligrino, Director for the Advanced Study of Ethics at Georgetown University, and Dr. George Lundberg, Editor of the Journal of the American Medical Association, also participated in its development. Dr. Roger Bulger, President of the Association of Academic Health Centers, and Dr. Ralph Crashaw, a practicing psychiatrist in Oregon, who has been active locally and nationally in ethical issues that pertain to physicians, were also co-authors. Finally, Dr. Lonnie Bristow, the President of the American Medical Association, and Dr. Jeremiah Barondess, the President of the New York Academy of Medicine, are authors.

As with the other foundational biomedical ethical principles, the ethical duty of nonmaleficence applies to omissions (i.e., the failure to act when one should act), as well as to affirmative acts. For example, the malicious, intentional abandonment of a patient by a treating health care provider constitutes a breach of the duty not to intentionally harm the abandoned patient.

Another example of a breach of the ethical principle of nonmaleficence involves the situation in which a health care provider engages in sexual relations—nonconsensual or consensual—with a patient under his or her care. A patient may display transference emotions that are romantic in nature toward a health care provider; however, the provider breaches the ethical duties of nonmaleficence and beneficence when he or she allows countertransference emotions to convert the professional relationship into a personal and intimate one.

Justice. **Justice** equates to equity, or fair treatment. As it relates to the official conduct of health care professionals, justice involves comporting oneself in a way so as to maximize fairness toward all patients and potential patients requiring intervention by the provider. The concept of justice applies not only to health care professionals as individuals but to specific health care disciplines and organizations and, more broadly, to health care delivery.

Distributive justice is concerned with how equitably health care services are distributed at the macro or societal level. Distributive justice issues include, among others, political debate over universal health insurance coverage, Medicare eligibility for patients with end-stage renal disease requiring kidney dialysis, prevention and treatment of patients with acquired immunodeficiency syndrome (AIDS) and other catastrophic diseases, and the rationing of health care interventions near the end of life.

Comparative justice addresses how health care is delivered at the micro or individual level. Comparative justice issues include, among many others, reimbursement and denial of care issues involving individual patients and the disparate treatment of patients on the basis of age, disability, gender, race and ethnicity, or religion. The Tuskegee Syphilis Study, conducted from 1932 to 1972, is an example of a comparative justice breach of professional ethics. In this study, 400 African-American men with syphilis were denied life-saving treatment (i.e., penicillin, after its discovery and release in the 1940s) so that researchers could study the effects of the disease. Publicity about this and other medical research studies led to the publication of the Belmont Report[18] and the promulgation of formal federal (and state and institutional) guidelines concerning the ethical treatment of human research subjects. On May 16, 1997, President Bill Clinton publicly apologized on behalf of the federal government in a White House ceremony to four of eight survivors of this ghoulish experiment.[19,20] Consider the following clinical practice dilemma:

The concept of justice applies not only to health care professionals as individuals but to specific health care disciplines and organizations and, more broadly, to health care delivery.

D, an emergency room physician, examines P, a patient who complains of severe abdominal cramping and pain. Fearing a possible bowel obstruction, D requests permission from X, a physician managed care gatekeeper, to admit P for tests. X denies the request, based on a diagnostic algorithm developed and used by the managed care organization to determine whether to admit patients with specified symptoms. D strongly believes that P should be admitted. What should D do?

D has established a professional relationship with P and has the legal and ethical duty to take whatever action is necessary to act in the patient's best medical interests, including admitting him irrespective of the reimbursement consequences of the admission. Fulfilling this duty may place D at risk of loss of employment or reinstatement with the managed care organization; however, D's higher legal and ethical duty is owed to P. To send P home might constitute a breach of professional ethics and intentional abandonment under these circumstances. Neither the law nor standards of professional ethics have changed significantly to accommodate the business of managed care.

Health practitioners are not the only professionals who face economic or other risks for "doing the right thing." Other professionals also encounter personal risks incident to fulfilling their professional duties. Consider the newspaper reporter who is jailed for refusing to violate the ethical duty not to reveal a confidential source to a judge or lawyer in a deposition, or the police, military, or fire professional who makes the ultimate sacrifice of his or her life in the line of duty.

A federal law related to the foundational biomedical ethical principle of individual justice is the Emergency Medical Treatment and Active Labor Act of 1986,[21] (EMTALA) or the federal "antidumping law." This law was enacted largely in response to well-publicized instances of indigent patient transfers to charity facilities by for-profit hospitals wishing to avoid a financial loss incident to their care.

EMTALA applies to all hospitals receiving federal funding for patient care. The law mandates that these facilities conduct medical screening examinations on all emergent patients and on all female patients in active labor, as well as stabilize bona fide emergency patients before transferring them to other (charity) facilities, without regard for the patients' ability to pay. EMTALA was intended to augment the ethical and common law duties on the part of hospitals to care for indigent emergency patients and patients in active labor and to create a uniform national standard to replace the scant number of inconsistent state laws concerning patient dumping.

Autonomy. **Autonomy** means *self-governance.* Respect for autonomy is based on respect for individual self-determination. In the health care delivery system,

---

The law mandates that...facilities conduct medical screening examinations on all emergent patients and on all female patients in active labor, as well as stabilize bona fide emergency patients before transferring them to other (charity) facilities, without regard for the patients' ability to pay.

18

patients and research subjects have the right to control what is done for or to them, respectively. For patients, autonomy rights exist whether or not the patient pays for care. For research subjects, the right of control over the intervention applies irrespective of the existence or amount of compensation. (The rights and protection of human research subjects is discussed further in Chapter 9.)

Health care professionals also exercise autonomy rights. They exercise control over physical facilities, assistants and other support personnel acting under supervision, equipment, and over the evaluative, diagnostic, and intervention processes within the applicable scope of professional practice.

Patient autonomy: the concept of self-determination. Patient autonomy rights are prominently reflected in modern-day laws and in the customary practices governing health care delivery. These laws and customs mandate, in part, strong and active patient involvement in interventional decision making. Health care organizations and professionals came to universally recognize in the twentieth century the right of patients to be involved in, and ultimately to control, treatment decision making processes.

This patient autonomy right of involvement and ultimate control over treatment is reflected in documents found in most or all hospitals describing patient rights and responsibilities incident to care. An excellent example of such a document is Brooke Army Medical Center's Patients' Bill of Rights and Responsibilities (Boxes 1-4 and 1-5),[22] modeled after the American Hospital Association's Patient Bill of Rights.[23]

Box 1-4. Patients' Rights

As a patient receiving care in this hospital, you have the right to:

- Considerate and respectful services.
- Privacy, including the right to request a chaperone.
- Confidentiality.
- Know which doctor/healthcare provider is primarily responsible for your care.
- Be spoken to in a language that is understandable.
- Be informed of hospital policies and regulations.
- Make advance medical directives (living wills and/or appoint a person to make health care decisions for you).
- Healthcare which recognizes your personal values, cultural practices and spiritual beliefs.
- Participate in decisions involving your healthcare.
- Clear, concise explanations of all proposed treatments, procedures, operations and risks.
- Current and complete information about your diagnosis, treatment and expected results.

Continued

Box 1-4. Patients' Rights—cont'd

- Refuse treatment (to the extent permitted by law and government regulations).
- Know the identity and professional status of individuals providing services.
- Be informed of (and elect not to participate in) any human research or other experimentation projects affecting your care.
- See the clinic or ward supervisor (Officer in Charge) or the Patient Representative to voice concerns, complaints, compliments and/or make recommendations for improvement.*

Box 1-5. Patients' Responsibilities

We consider you a partner in your healthcare. In order to provide you with the best possible care, we would like to request that you:

- Follow all hospital policies and procedures.
- Provide accurate and complete information about your health and medical condition.
- Ask for more information if you do not understand your illness or treatment.
- Follow the treatment plan that you and the doctor/healthcare provider responsible for your care agree upon and report any unexpected changes in your condition.
- Keep scheduled appointments, or give proper notice to the clinic or Patient Appointment System.
- Fully disclose your health insurance and liability insurance policies, and/or assure that financial obligations for your healthcare are fulfilled as promptly as possible.
- Respect the rights of other patients, families, visitors and staff.
- Respect the property of other persons and of the hospital.*

A patient's right of autonomy also includes the right to refuse treatment, after all reasonable options and the consequences of refusal of treatment have been explained to the patient. Is the patient's right to refuse intervention absolute? No. Courts have ruled on occasion that treatment may be given compulsorily to patients under special circumstances, such as when the life of a third party (e.g., fetus carried by a mother) is at risk if treatment is not provided to the patient. More and more, however, courts are ruling in ways that evince greater respect for patient autonomy, irrespective of the consequences of patient decisions to innocent third parties. (This topic is addressed in greater detail in Chapter 9: Life and Death Decision Making.)

Finally, it is universally recognized that patients have the right to choose their own health care providers. Laws in all states and professional ethics codes recognize this inherent patient right. For example, Section 3.3, Provision of

*From *Patients' bill of rights and responsibilities*, BAMC Handout 002-97, Brooke Army Medical Center, Fort Sam Houston, Texas, 1997.

Services, of the American Physical Therapy Association's *Guide for Professional Conduct* [24] reads:

> Physical therapists shall recognize the individual's freedom of choice in selection of physical therapy services.

Autonomy for health care professionals: the concept of self-governance. Health care professionals enjoy a domain of autonomous professional practice that has been granted to them, in part, through licensure laws and certification processes and, in part, through customary practices. In all disciplines, health professionals must maintain the ability to exercise independent judgment within their domains of health professional practice. Again, by way of example, Section 3.1, Acceptance of Responsibility of the American Physical Therapy Association's *Guide for Professional Conduct* [25] requires that:

> Regardless of practice setting, physical therapists shall maintain the ability to make independent judgments.

Managed care and health care reform initiatives have the potential to adversely affect professional autonomy in a number of ways. A draft version of the 1993 federal health reform initiative would have given regional health alliances broad authority to supervene certification and state licensure restrictions on professional practice in unspecified ways. Managed care contractual alliances may create barriers to participation for providers not part of a preferred provider network. Managed care restrictions on provider-patient communication in the form of contractual "gag clauses" and on parameters of practice also derogate from health care professional autonomy and therefore must, because of their potential adverse impact on patient care delivery, be addressed by the health professional, political, consumer, and other relevant communities.

Systems Approach to Health Care Professional Ethical Decision Making

Health care ethical decision making, whether in clinical, educational, research, school, home, or other settings, requires careful compliance with professional and, where applicable, institutional ethical standards and with legal mandates. As with legal requirements, ignorance of ethical responsibilities is no excuse for noncompliance.

There are several recognized frameworks for ethical decision making for health care professionals.[26,27,28,29] Ethical decision-making models governing patient care are based on the foundational biomedical ethical principles of beneficence, nonmaleficence, autonomy, and justice, and are reflective of core professional attributes and duties, including altruism, competency, confidentiality, fidelity, and

The four foundational biomedical ethical principles guiding the official conduct of health care professionals are beneficence, nonmaleficence, justice, and autonomy.

21

truthfulness, among others. Conducting oneself in conformity with these principles, attributes, and duties is seemingly more difficult under the current managed care paradigm, which poses significant actual and potential conflicts of interest. Most analytical ethical decision-making models have common core elements:

- Identification of a problem, issue, or dilemma having ethical implications
- Identification of relevant facts and unknowns and formulation of reasonable assumptions about the problem, issue, or dilemma
- Delineation and analysis of viable courses of action to resolve the problem, issue, or dilemma
- Selection of an option for implementation based on an appropriate ethics approach and ethical guidelines and in conformity with controlling ethical and legal directives.

Ignorance of one's professional ethical responsibilities is no excuse for noncompliance.

The systems approach augments this model with a feedback loop. Under the systems approach, a decision maker carefully monitors and obtains feedback on a chosen course of action for appropriateness, efficacy, and effectiveness—on an ongoing basis—and modifies the chosen course of action (or rejects it outright and substitutes another course of action) if, on the basis of negative feedback, it is adjudged not to be optimal. For more information on general systems theory and thinking, see von Bertalanffy's *General Systems Theory: Foundations, Development, Application*.[30]

Von Bertalanffy developed systems theory in the 1920s. Today, it is widely used in engineering, the natural sciences, and business and management.

Under the systems approach to health care professional ethical decision making, a decision maker must evaluate and reevaluate a myriad of factors relevant to a problem, issue, or dilemma at all steps of the analysis. These factors include, among others:

- **S**ociocultural considerations, such as gender, race and ethnicity, religion, sexual preference, and other factors, as they apply to a problem, issue, or dilemma
- **L**egal implications associated with a decision
- **E**thical imperatives (i.e., Will the decision maker's conduct conform to a governing professional code of ethics or with the decision maker's personal morals and ethical standards?)
- **E**conomic impact of a course of action on those persons affected by its implementation
- **P**olitical ramifications associated with a course of action

In addition to applying these **S-L-E-E-P**[31] factors, a decision maker should also always apply the principle of symmetry[32] to the resolution of a health care

ethical problem, issue, or dilemma within the systems approach to health care professional ethical decision making. The principle of symmetry provides a 180-degree
analysis of a chosen course of action. It requires a decision maker to analyze a decision by taking the opposing point of view and analyzing its implementation from that
perspective.

Figure 1-4 depicts a circular flow diagram of the systems approach to
health care professional ethical decision making.

Summary

Health care professionals must comply with their own personal moral beliefs, the civil
and criminal laws of the jurisdiction in which they practice, and the professional
ethics standards of their professional associations and other entities. Occasionally,
these governing directives are in conflict, creating serious dilemmas for health professionals and patients under their care.

There are four foundational biomedical ethical concepts affecting health
care professional ethics. *Beneficence* involves acting in a patient's best interests.
Health care professionals are their patients' fiduciaries (i.e., they stand in a position of
special trust and confidence). *Nonmaleficence* means that health care professionals are

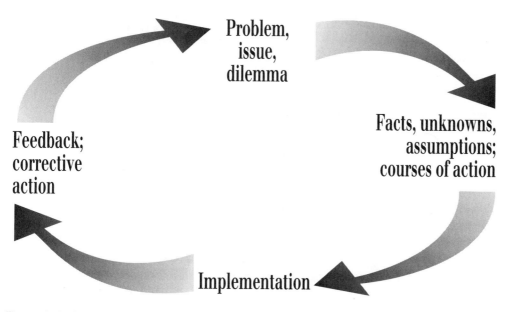

Figure 1-4. Systems approach to health care professional ethical decision making.

23

bound not to intentionally harm patients under their care. *Justice* involves equitable treatment of all patients. *Autonomy* evidences respect for patients' inherent right of self-determination—particularly in controlling treatment decision making. The implementation of these guiding principles—particularly beneficence, justice, and autonomy—has been made more difficult under managed care, in which the interests of provider and payer interests are often in conflict with patient needs or desires.

Health care professionals must employ a systematic approach to health care professional ethical decision making. The systems approach contains the following elements: (1) identification of a problem, issue, or dilemma with ethical implications; (2) identification of relevant facts and unknowns, and formulation of reasonable assumptions; (3) delineation and analysis of viable courses of action; (4) implementation of a course of action; and (5) monitoring and modification (if necessary) of an executed course of action, based on ongoing feedback.

Cases and Questions

1. Develop a draft version of a model patient code of ethical conduct, applicable to patients in rehabilitation settings. Highlight only the main areas of coverage under the model code.

2. Consider the following clinical practice problem:

   A physical therapist in private practice in a large metropolitan area in the northeastern United States is contemplating the establishment of a pro bono publico (reduced or no fee) service within her practice for indigent patients needing her services. Analyze the problem under the systems approach to health care professional ethical decision making.

Suggested Answers for Cases and Questions

1. A patient code of ethics may contain the following provisions (among possible others):

   ### Model Rehabilitation Patient Code of Ethics

   A patient in the rehabilitation setting is expected to:
   I. Provide accurate and complete information to a primary health care provider or other rehabilitation professional, relevant to a consultation or treatment.
   II. Listen carefully to information provided by a health care provider; ask relevant questions about recommended interventions; and make a knowing, intelligent, voluntary, and unequivocal decision to accept or decline a recommended intervention.

Suggested Answers for Cases and Questions—cont'd

   III. Respect the rights and dignity of all other persons in the health care setting, and respect the property of others.

   IV. Cooperate with evaluating and treating health care professionals to the maximum extent feasible, and ask relevant questions about care interventions throughout the process of care delivery.

   V. Conduct himself or herself in such a way as to maintain an appropriate patient–health care professional relationship with his or her providers.

2. Factors for analysis under the systems approach to health care professional ethical decision making:

- Problem. There are a significant number of patients requiring physical therapy services in the community who present themselves in this clinic for care, lacking the ability to pay for those services.
- Facts, unknowns, and assumptions. One sample factor is given for each category. Others may also apply.
  - Sociocultural considerations. Indigent patients presenting in this clinic for care are disproportionately working mothers and their children.
  - Legal implications. It is assumed that the state permits indigent patients to sign a waiver of liability for simple negligence incident to no-fee health care.
  - Ethical imperatives. According to Principle 8, Section 8.1 of APTA's Guide for Professional Conduct:
    - **8.1 Pro Bono Service**
      Physical therapists should render *pro bono* publico (reduced or no fee) services to patients lacking the ability to pay for services, as each physical therapist's practice permits.
  - Economic impact. Accepting a fixed number of *pro bono* patients for care (e.g., three patients at any one time) is not expected to adversely affect the profitability of the practice.
  - Political ramifications. Establishing a *pro bono publico* policy and publicizing it will enhance the business goodwill of the practice.
- Courses of action:
  1. Do not accept any *pro bono* patients in the clinic, except as required by law.
  2. Accept up to three *pro bono* patients (based on demonstrated need) in the clinic's practice mix at any one time.
- Option for implementation. Accept up to three *pro bono* patients (based on demonstrated need) in the clinic's practice mix at any one time.
- Feedback. Monitor the option implemented for appropriateness, efficacy, and effectiveness; modify or discontinue, as necessary.

References

1. Walton CC: *The moral manager,* Cambridge, Mass, 1988, Ballinger Publishing.

2. Nadien V: Shevardnadze sacrifices diplomat for $30 million. In *Current digest of the post-Soviet press* 49:2,24, Feb 1997.

3. *Griswold v. Connecticut,* 381 US 479, 1965.

4. Cleverley WO: *Essentials of health care finance,* ed 4, Gaithersburg, Md, 1997, Aspen Publishers.

5. Fleming MH, Johnson JA, Marina M, Spergel EL, Townsend B: *Occupational therapy: directions for the future,* Bethesda, Md, 1987, AOTA.

6. Richardson ML, White KK: *Ethics applied,* New York, 1993, McGraw-Hill.

7. Bailey DM, Schwartzberg SL: *Ethical and legal dilemmas in occupational therapy,* Philadelphia, 1995, FA Davis.

8. Jonsen AR, Siegler M, Winslade WJ: *Clinical ethics,* ed 3, New York, 1992, McGraw-Hill.

9. La Puma J: Clinical ethics, mission, and vision: practical wisdom in health care. In *Hospitals & health care administration* 35(3):321, 1990.

10. Davis N: *Courts statistics project,* 1994, Personal communication.

11. American Physical Therapy Association: *Guide for professional conduct,* Alexandria, 1997, APTA.

12. Fletcher J: *Situational ethics: the new morality,* Philadelphia, 1966, Westminster Press.

13. American Occupational Therapy Association: *Occupational therapy code of ethics,* Bethesda, Md, 1994, AOTA.

14. Richardson: Note 6, 732.

15. Beauchamp TL, Childress JF: *Principles of biomedical ethics,* ed 4, New York, 1994, Oxford University Press.

16. Pelligrino ED: The metamorphosis of medical ethics: a 30-year retrospective, *JAMA* 269:1158, 1993.

17. Patient-Physician Covenant.

18. National Commission for the Protection of Human Subjects of Biomedical and Behavioral Research: *Belmont report: ethical principles and guidelines for the protection of human subjects of research,* Washington, DC, 1978, US Government Printing Office.

19. Beck J: Apology for syphilis project overdue. In *Indianapolis Star,* May 18, 1997, D2.

20. Kasindorf M: Tuskegee survivors make trek to capital for apology. In *USA Today,* May 15, 1997, 6A.

21. The Emergency Medical Treatment and Active Labor Act of 1986, 42 United States Code Section 1395dd.

22. *Patients' Bill of Rights and Responsibilities,* San Antonio, 1997, Brooke Army Medical Center Quality Improvement Committee.

23. Patient Bill of Rights, Chicago, 1992, American Hospital Association.

24. *Guide,* note 11, principle 3, section 3.3A.

25. *Ibid,* Section 3.1C.

26. Anderson GR, Glesnes-Anderson VA: *Health care ethics: a guide for decision makers,* Gaithersburg Md, 1987, Aspen Publishers.

27. Kyler P: *Everyday ethics: common concerns in occupational therapy,* Rockville Md, 1995, AOTA.

28. Purtilo R: *Ethical dimensions in the health professions,* ed 2, Philadelphia, 1993, WB Saunders.

29. Richardson, note 6, 54.

30. von Bertalanffy L: *General systems theory: foundations, development, application,* New York, 1968, George Braziller.

31. Adapted from Dr. William Moore, Jr, Professor, The University of Texas at Austin: *Ethics and values* graduate course, EDA 388V, Spring 1997. Used with permission.

32. *Ibid.*

Suggested Readings

Anderson GR, Glesnes-Anderson VA: *Health care ethics: a guide for decision makers,* Gaithersburg Md, 1987, Aspen Publishers.

Bailey DM, Schwartzberg SL: *Ethical and legal dilemmas in occupational therapy,* Philadelphia, 1995, FA Davis.

Beauchamp TL, Childress JF: *Principles of biomedical ethics,* ed 4, New York, 1994, Oxford University Press.

Cleverley WO: *Essentials of health care finance,* ed 4, Gaithersburg, Md, 1997, Aspen Publishers.

Fleming MH, Johnson JA, Marina M, Spergel EL, Townsend B: *Occupational therapy: directions for the future,* Bethesda, Md, 1987, AOTA.

Fletcher J: *Situational ethics: the new morality,* Philadelphia, 1966, Westminster Press.

Hoffman WM, Moore JM: *Business ethics,* ed 2, New York, 1990, McGraw-Hill.

Jonsen AR, Siegler M, Winslade WJ: *Clinical ethics,* ed 3, New York, 1992, McGraw-Hill.

Kyler P: *Everyday ethics: common concerns in occupational therapy,* Rockville Md, 1995, AOTA.

La Puma J: Clinical ethics, mission, and vision: practical wisdom in health care. In *Hospitals & health care administration* 35(3):321, 1990.

National Commission for the Protection of Human Subjects of Biomedical and Behavioral Research: *Belmont report: ethical principles and guidelines for the protection of human subjects of research,* Washington, DC, 1978, US Government Printing Office.

Patient Bill of Rights, Chicago, 1992, American Hospital Association.

Pelligrino ED: The metamorphosis of medical ethics: a 30-year retrospective, *JAMA* 269:1158, 1993.

Purtilo R: *Ethical dimensions in the health professions,* ed 2, Philadelphia, 1993, WB Saunders.

Richardson ML, White KK: *Ethics applied,* New York, 1993, McGraw-Hill.

The Emergency Medical Treatment and Active Labor Act of 1986, 42 United States Code Section 1395dd.

von Bertalanffy L: *General systems theory: foundations, development, application,* New York, 1968, George Braziller.

Walton CC: *The moral manager,* Cambridge, Mass, 1988, Ballinger Publishing.

Codification of Ethical Duties

This chapter describes the purposes of professional codes of ethics and examines the ethics codes for occupational therapy, orthotics and prosthetics, physical therapy, rehabilitation nursing, respiratory therapy, and the speech-language-hearing professions. The nature of directive and nondirective ethical provisions within ethics codes is explored. The chapter overviews the complaint, disciplinary, and appeal processes for the professions of physical and occupational therapy and orthotics and prosthetics, as representative of processes for other rehabilitation and health professions. The chapter concludes with discussion of the oversight and adjudicatory roles of state agencies and the courts.

●

Purposes of Professional Codes of Ethics

Professional codes of ethics have four coprimary purposes.[1] First, a professional code of ethics is **directive,** that is, it provides guidance for mandatory behavior by members of a profession. (Professional ethics codes may also provide nondirective guidance for recommended conduct of members of a profession.) Second, a code must be **protective** of the rights of patients, clients, and subjects; their significant others; and the public at large. Third, a professional code of ethics must be **specific,** that is, it must address areas of ethical problems, issues, and dilemmas particular to the discipline(s) governed by the code. Finally, a professional ethics code must be **enforceable** and **enforced.**

The codes of ethics for the professions of occupational therapy, orthotics and prosthetics, physical therapy, rehabilitation nursing, respiratory therapy, and speech-language-hearing professionals are reprinted in the appendixes.

Roles and Responsibilities in Developing Ethical Principles and Enforcing Compliance

Every health care professional discipline (through its professional association[s]) has a code of ethics in place governing the official conduct of its members. This section examines in great detail the ethics codes for the professions of physical and occupational therapy and orthotics and prosthetics. Readers are urged to conduct a comparative analysis of these professional codes of ethics and the ethics codes for other rehabilitation and health professions.

Standards

Codes of ethics may contain two general types of provisions: directive and nondirective. Directive provisions address required conduct. Nondirective provisions are of two types, addressing permissive conduct and recommended conduct. Directive provisions normally contain the action verbs "shall," "will," "must," "required," "responsible," or, in the negative, "may not," "shall not," or "will not." Nondirective provisions addressing permissive conduct may contain the action verbs "may" or "are not prohibited from...," whereas nondirective provisions addressing recommended conduct typically contain the action verbs "should" or "should not." Examples of directive and nondirective ethics provisions from the American Physical Therapy Association's Guide for Professional Conduct are:

● **Directive:** Physical therapists *shall* [emphasis added] recognize that each individual is different from all other individuals and shall respect and be responsive to those differences.[2]

Codes of ethics may contain two general types of provisions: directive and nondirective. Directive provisions address required conduct. Nondirective provisions address permissive and recommended conduct.

● **Nondirective (permissive conduct):** Physical therapists *may* [emphasis added] enter into agreements with organizations to provide physical therapy services if such agreements do not violate the ethical principles of the Association.[3]

● **Nondirective (recommended conduct):** Physical therapists *should* [emphasis added] render *pro bono publico* (reduced or no fee) services to patients lacking the ability to pay for services, as each physical therapist's practice permits.[4]

The provisions in the Occupational Therapy Code of Ethics are not differentiated into directive and nondirective components. All of the ethical principles in the Occupational Therapy Code of Ethics are directive, and all contain the action verb "shall." For example, Principle 2A states that:

> Occupational therapy personnel *shall* collaborate with service recipients or their surrogate(s) in determining goals and priorities throughout the intervention process.

The Canons of Ethical Conduct governing the official conduct of certified orthotists and prosthetists contains both directive and nondirective provisions. Examples of directive provisions within the Canons include the following:

> The orthotist or prosthetist *must* [emphasis added] receive a prescription from a physician or appropriately licensed health care provider before providing any orthosis or prosthesis to a patient. The prescription must state that the patient is ready for orthotic or prosthetic management. It is the responsibility of the physician or appropriately licensed health care provider, and not the orthotist or prosthetist, to determine the medical appropriateness of the orthosis or prosthesis.[5]
>
> All orthotists and prosthetists *shall* [emphasis added] provide competent services and shall use all efforts to meet the patient's orthotic and prosthetic requirements. Upon accepting an individual for orthotic or prosthetic services, the orthotist or prosthetist *shall* assume the responsibility for evaluating that individual; planning, implementing and supervising the patient; reevaluating and changing the program; and maintaining adequate records of the case, including progress reports.[6]

Examples of nondirective provisions within the Canons (within mixed nondirective-directive Canon provisions) include the following:

● **Nondirective (permissive conduct):** The orthotist or prosthetist *may* [emphasis added] repair or adjust an orthosis or prosthesis without notifying the prescribing health care provider. However, such repairs or adjustments must conform to the original prescription. Any repairs, adjustments, modifications, and/or replacements that substantially alter the original prescription must be authorized by the physician or the prescribing health care provider.[7]

● **Nondirective (recommended conduct):** The orthotist or prosthetist *should* exercise appropriate respect for other health care professionals. Concerns regarding patient care provided by other professionals *should* [emphasis added] be addressed directly to that professional, rather than to the patient. In the event that such concerns rise to the level of criminal violation, incompetency, malpractice, or a violation of these Canons, then the orthotist or prosthetist must immediately notify the American Board for Certification in Orthotic and Prosthetics (ABC). The Committee will take appropriate action in accordance with these Canons and applicable law.[8]

Frameworks for Selected Rehabilitation Health Care Professional Codes of Ethics

Physical Therapy

Physical Therapists. The American Physical Therapy Association's Code of Ethics and implementing Guide for Professional Conduct contain both directive and nondirective ethical provisions regulating the official conduct of member physical therapists. The framework of the Guide for Professional Conduct is as follows:

Principle 1 (Respect for Rights and Dignity)
 1.1: Attitudes
 1.2: Confidentiality
 1.3: Patient Relations
 1.4: Informed Consent
Principle 2 (Compliance with Laws and Regulations)
 2.1: Professional Practice
Principle 3 (Responsibility, Professional Autonomy)
 3.1: Responsibility
 3.2: Delegation
 3.3: Provision of Services
 3.4: Referral Relationships
 3.5: Practice Arrangements
Principle 4 (Standards: Maintenance, Promotion)
 4.1: Continuing Education
 4.2: Review and Self-Assessment
 4.3: Research
 4.4: Education
Principle 5 (Renumeration)
 5.1: Fiscally Sound Renumeration

5.2: Business Practices/Fee Arrangements
5.3: Endorsement of Equipment or Services
5.4: Gifts
Principle 6 (Professional Information Dissemination)
6.1: Information About the Profession
6.2: Information About Services
Principle 7 (Professional Responsibility)
7.1: Consumer Protection
7.2: Disclosure of Potential Conflicts of Interest
Principle 8 (Public Health)
8.1: *Pro Bono* Service

Physical Therapist Assistants. The American Physical Therapy
Association's Standards of Ethical Conduct for the Physical Therapist Assistant and
implementing Guide for Conduct of the Affiliate Member, regulating the official conduct of member physical therapist assistants also contain directive and nondirective
provisions. The framework of the Guide for Conduct of the Affiliate Member is as
follows:

Standard 1 (Performance of Services Under Supervision)
1.1 Supervisory Relationships
1.2 Performance of Services
Standard 2 (Respect for Rights and Dignity)
2.1 Attitudes
2.2 Requests for Release of Information
2.3 Protection of Privacy
2.4 Patient Relations
Standard 3 (Standards: Maintenance, Promotion)
3.1 Information About Services
3.2 Organizational Equipment
3.3 Endorsement of Equipment
3.4 Financial Considerations
3.5 Exploitation of Patients
Standard 4 (Compliance with Law)
4.1 Supervisory Relationships
4.2 Representation
Standard 5 (Exercise of Judgment)
5.1 Patient Treatment
5.2 Patient Safety
5.3 Qualifications
5.4 Discontinuance of Treatment Programs

        5.5 Continuing Education

     Standard 6 (Professional Responsibility)

        6.1 Consumer Protection

All but four of the standards and their sections in the Guide for Conduct of the Affiliate Member are directive in nature. Those four nondirective provisions are all of the permissive type.

Occupational Therapy

The American Occupational Therapy Association's unitary Occupational Therapy Code of Ethics is intended to be all-inclusive, binding *all* occupational therapy practitioners who are members of the professional Association to its provisions. Its framework is as follows:

     Principle 1 (Beneficence)
        A. Equitable provision of services
        B. Professional relationships
        C. Avoidance of harm to recipients of services
        D. Reasonableness of fees (23)

     Principle 2 (Respect for Rights of Service Recipients)
        A. Continuous collaboration on goals and priorities
        B. Patient informed consent
        C. Research subject informed consent
        D. Right to refuse services or participation
        E. Confidentiality

     Principle 3 (Competence)
        A. Credentials
        B. Standards of practice
        C. Professional development
        D. Accurate and current information
        E. Appropriate delegation
        F. Appropriate supervision
        G. Referral, consultation

     Principle 4 (Compliance with Laws and Policies)
        A. Personal compliance
        B. Communication of legal and administrative duties
        C. Compliance by those under supervision
        D. Accurate documentation and communication

     Principle 5 (Accuracy in Information About Services)
        A. Personal representation
        B. Actual and potential conflicts of interests
        C. False, deceptive, unfair communications

Principle 6 (Professional Relations)
A. Confidentiality
B. Representation of qualifications
C. Reporting of breaches of ethics

Orthotics and Prosthetics

The Canons of Ethical Conduct, promulgated by the American Board for Certification in Orthotics and Prosthetics, is binding on certified orthotists and prosthetists, facilities providing orthotic and prosthetic services that are accredited by the American Board for Certification in Orthotics and Prosthetics, and orthotic and prosthetic assistants and technicians. Its framework is as follows:

I. Preamble
    Canon 1.1: Introduction
    Canon 1.2: Ethics, Custom and the Law
II. Practitioner Responsibilities to the Physician
    Canon 2.1: Diagnosis and Prescription
    Canon 2.2: Orthosis and Prosthesis Evaluation and Recommendation
    Canon 2.3: Changes in Patient's Condition
    Canon 2.4: Provision of Service
    Canon 2.5: Altering Orthosis or Prosthesis
III. Responsibilities to the Patient
    Canon 3.1: Confidential Information
    Canon 3.2: Competency
    Canon 3.3: Research
    Canon 3.4: Trust and Honesty
    Canon 3.5: Fees and Compensation
    Canon 3.6: Practice Arrangements
    Canon 3.7: Delay in Services
    Canon 3.8: Compliance with Laws and Regulations
    Canon 3.9: Consumer Protection
    Canon 3.10: Delegation of Responsibility
    Canon 3.11: Information to Patient
    Canon 3.12: Illegal Discrimination
IV. Responsibilities to Colleagues and the Profession
    Canon 4.1: Dignity and Status
    Canon 4.2: Commercialism
    Canon 4.3: Solicitation
    Canon 4.4: Peer Review
    Canon 4.5: Education

Enforcement of Ethics Codes: Disciplinary Processes

Health professional ethical standards are enforced by professional associations, credentialing bodies, and state licensure or regulatory administrative agencies. These ethical provisions are also indirectly enforced by the courts in civil and criminal proceedings in which violations of professional ethics also constitute violations of the law.

      The jurisdictional models and procedural processes for physical and occupational therapy and orthotics and prosthetics are presented in this section. Readers are invited to research the ethical jurisdiction, complaint, adjudication, and appeal processes for their respective professions, and compare them with those in place for these professions.

Participants and Processes

Physical Therapy

The American Physical Therapy Association has ethical jurisdiction over the more than 60,000 physical therapists and physical therapist assistants who are members of the Association.[9] A written complaint of unethical conduct on the part of a member physical therapist or physical therapist assistant is the starting point for an initiation of investigation and disciplinary action, pursuant to the Procedural Document on Disciplinary Action of the American Physical Therapy Association.[10]

      A complaint can be made by anyone having knowledge (first-hand or otherwise) of a suspected ethical violation by an Association member. The signed, written complaint is forwarded to the state Chapter President who: (1) forwards an informational copy of the complaint to the Judicial Committee, and (2) makes an initial determination as to whether the complaint is actionable. Acknowledgment of receipt of the complaint must be forwarded to the **complainant** by the Chapter President within 15 days of receipt. Along with acknowledgment, the Chapter President advises the complainant that the **respondent** may have the right to learn the complainant's identity.

A written complaint of unethical conduct on the part of an Association member can be made by anyone having knowledge (first-hand or otherwise) of a suspected ethical violation.

If a complaint is nonactionable because an allegation does not involve a violation of the Code of Ethics or Standards of Ethical Conduct, or, if in the judgment of the Chapter President, the allegation does not warrant action, the complaint is dismissed by the Chapter President. If the complaint is actionable, the respondent member is notified of the charge(s) and of the specific provisions of the Code or Standards allegedly violated.

A Chapter President may initiate action on his or her own (without a written complaint), based on public information. Proof of commission of a crime related to a member's professional status, or of a felony, or of revocation of licensure, is *prima facie* (presumed) evidence of an actionable ethics violation and triggers interim suspension of membership until Judicial Committee action at its next regularly scheduled semiannual meeting.

In all other actionable cases, the Chapter President forwards the case file to the Chapter Ethics Committee (CEC) for processing. The CEC either summarily dismisses charges, based on available evidence, or appoints an investigator, who conducts a comprehensive, unbiased investigation of the charges against the respondent; compiles an investigative file; and makes findings of fact (but not conclusions or recommendations).

If the CEC determines that charges against a respondent are unsubstantiated, the CEC may summarily dismiss the complaint, under which option the respondent does not have the right to learn the name of the complainant. Otherwise, the respondent is notified of his or her right to a copy of the investigative file and to a hearing of the charges.

With or without a hearing, the CEC makes specific conclusions and recommendations on charges against a respondent, which must be either dismissal of the charges or disciplinary action by the Judicial Committee. Judicial Committee disciplinary actions include written reprimand, membership probation (from 6 months to 2 years), membership suspension (1 year or longer), or expulsion from the Association.

Once properly notified of the CEC recommendations, a respondent has the right to request a hearing before the Judicial Committee at its next semiannual meeting in Alexandria, Virginia. At this hearing, as at the state level, the respondent may be accompanied by an attorney, who serves as a silent advisor to the respondent during the proceedings.

With or without another hearing, the Judicial Committee takes action on a complaint as follows: the Judicial Committee may adopt the disciplinary recommendation(s) of the CEC, dismiss charges or award a less severe disciplinary sanction, or **remand** the case to the CEC for further action.

After appropriate notification, a respondent has the right to appeal the Judicial Committee's decision to the Board of Directors within 30 days. The Board of Directors may affirm the decision of the Judicial Committee, dismiss charges or impose a less severe disciplinary sanction, or remand the case to the Judicial

Committee for further action. Once final, publication of disciplinary action takes place in the Association's publications of general circulation. Published information is limited to the name of the respondent, the disciplinary action taken, and the effective date of the action. Beyond this summary information, the details of disciplinary proceedings are confidential, and further information about proceedings is not normally disseminated without a court order.

Occupational Therapy

American Occupational Therapy Association. The American Occupational Therapy Association has ethical jurisdiction over the more than 48,000 certified occupational therapists and occupational therapy assistants who are members of the Association.[11] The procedures for receiving, evaluating, and adjudicating ethical complaints against members of the American Occupational Therapy Association are analogous to those employed by the American Physical Therapy Association, with a few important differences.[12]

A complaint of an ethical violation against a member of the Association may be filed by anyone having knowledge of a suspected ethical violation by an Association member. A signed, written complaint is filed with the Standards and Ethics Commission (SEC), for which an appointed Investigation Committee conducts a preliminary investigation to determine whether there is substantial evidence of an ethical violation. The Investigation Committee is empowered to make findings and recommendations concerning suspected ethical violations. If such evidence is found to exist, the SEC may issue a formal charge, which it forwards to the President of the Association, who then appoints a Judicial Counsel to adjudicate the charge.

The ad hoc Judicial Counsel, comprised of three members of the Association, presides at a hearing on charges against the member and is represented by legal counsel. A respondent may also be represented by legal counsel at such a hearing.

A finding that a member has committed an ethical violation may result in the award of one of the following disciplinary sanctions: censure, membership suspension, or expulsion from the Association. A respondent is notified in certified written form of the Judicial Counsel's decision by the President of the Association.

A respondent may file a timely written appeal of a disciplinary action to the Executive Director of the Association. Such an appeal is heard by a three-member panel, comprised of the Vice-President, Secretary, and Treasurer of the Association. An appeals hearing may or may not take place at the discretion of the Appeals Panel. The decision of the Appeals Panel is final.

National Board for Certification in Occupational Therapy. The National Board for Certification in Occupational Therapy (NBCOT), formerly known as the American Occupational Therapy Certification Board, is the national nongovernmental agency responsible for certification and recertification of certified occupational therapists and occupational therapy assistants.[13] It has jurisdiction to investigate complaints and take disciplinary action against all NBCOT-certified (and eligible) certified occupational therapists and occupational therapy assistants. In addition to adjudicating ethical complaints, NBCOT investigates and takes action on complaints alleging incompetence and impairment on the part of occupational therapy professionals. Its Procedures for Disciplinary Action[14] incorporates procedures that are similar to those employed by the associations governing the occupational and physical therapy professions.

The spectrum of disciplinary sanctions that can be awarded by the NBCOT includes, in order of progressive severity:
- Formal written reprimand
- Public censure
- Compulsory community service
- Compulsory participation in remediation programs
- Suspension of certification to practice for a definite term
- Ineligibility for certification, either for a definite or indefinite term
- Revocation of certification

Similar to the American Occupational Therapy Association, NBCOT may issue advisory opinions on matters under its jurisdiction, similar to procedures used by the American Bar Association, which governs the ethical conduct of member attorneys. At the time of the writing of this book, the American Occupational Therapy Association and the NBCOT were engaged in litigation over whether to continue the usage of the designations *OTR* and *COTA*, for occupational therapist, registered and for certified occupational therapy assistant, respectively.[15]

Orthotics and Prosthetics

The Canons of Ethical Conduct governing orthotics and prosthetics professionals and accredited facilities are enforced by the Committee on Character and Fitness (CCF) of the ABC. The three appointed members of the CCF are former members of the American Board for Certification in Orthotics and Prosthetics, whose identities are not disclosed to member professionals of the Board. They are empowered to investigate allegations of unethical or otherwise unprofessional conduct by members. The CCF is not empowered to investigate or take action on purely "economic issues as they relate to legitimate marketplace competition."[16]

The disciplinary procedures of the CCF are similar to those used with physical and occupational therapists, except that the range of permissible sanctions after a finding of culpability is more variegated. A complaint may be filed by any aggrieved party with the CCF or initiated by the CCF, *sua sponte.* After notification of charges (including the identity of the complainant), an accused has 30 days to respond to allegations and request (or waive) a hearing before the CCF. Formal versus informal proceedings are at the option of the CCF. On a finding of culpability, possible recommended sanctions include:

- Cease and desist order
- Practice supervision
- Reprimand
- Censure
- Probation and practice monitoring
- Referral to professional association and/or certification or licensure authority
- Suspension of certification
- Request for relinquishment by respondent of certification
- Revocation of certification
- Referral to criminal authorities

A respondent has 30 days to appeal a CCF disciplinary recommendation to the American Board for Certification in Orthotics and Prosthetics, before which a respondent may request a hearing at his or her own expense. A final decision by the American Board for Certification in Orthotics and Prosthetics is considered to be a final administrative action.[17]

Actions by State Regulatory Agencies

In addition to adverse action by professional associations and certification entities, disciplinary action for ethical violations against health care professionals can be undertaken by state regulatory and licensure agencies. These entities are public bodies; consequently, all the federal and state constitutional safeguards and procedures that apply to state actions generally apply to their actions.

Health professional regulatory entities have jurisdiction over professionals privileged to practice in the state and over those who practice without proper credentials. They operate pursuant to a state's federal constitutional "police power" to make and enforce standards for public health and safety.[18]

Administrative procedures for adjudicating disciplinary complaints alleging ethics violations (of practice acts or professional codes) are similar to those used by private associations and boards, except that as public entities, state regulatory bodies must pay strict attention to procedural and substantive due process requirements. Disciplinary sanctions that may be awarded by public regulatory entities include, among other possible adverse actions, public censure, suspension, and revocation of licensure or practice privileges.

Administrative procedures undertaken by state regulatory and licensure agencies for adjudicating disciplinary complaints alleging ethics violations are similar to those used by private associations, except that state regulatory bodies must pay attention to procedural and substantive due process requirements.

39

Public censure means dissemination of offenses and disciplinary sanctions to the general public. As with news about other public figures, the public has the constitutional "right to know" about disciplinary actions taken by states against licensed or otherwise regulated health care professionals. Recent examples of public censure of health professionals by state regulatory agencies include license suspension or revocation for corporal punishment of a spouse, prostitution, and nonpayment of child support by a licensee.[19,20]

Private associations and boards adjudicating disciplinary actions against health care professionals may or may not communicate formally with state regulatory entities about their activities. The policies of the American Occupational Therapy Association and NBCOT are to communicate information about disciplinary actions taken against member professionals to state regulatory entities via the Disciplinary Action Information Exchange Network.[21] The policy of the American Board for Certification in Orthotics and Prosthetics is similar to that of the American Occupational Therapy Association and NBCOT, that is, it communicates the names of decertified certificants and violations of the rules or canons involved to professional associations, state certifying and licensure entities, and public agencies, as appropriate.[22] The policy of the American Physical Therapy Association is to not routinely communicate specific information about its disciplinary proceedings to state regulatory entities, without a statute, regulation, or court order requiring such communication.[23] Of course, the proceedings of state regulatory entities are normally available to private associations and individuals because they are public records.

Due Process and Judicial Oversight of Health Professional Associations

In adverse administrative disciplinary actions by state regulatory agencies against health professionals, the federal constitutional due process clause of the fourteenth amendment requires that these governmental agencies afford procedural and substantive due process to respondents. State constitutions, statutes, and case law may afford additional protections to respondents in these public fora.

Procedural due process means an adequate notice of an adverse action and a reasonable opportunity to be heard. In the case of adverse professional licensure actions, a reasonable opportunity to be heard is synonymous with the right to a hearing.

Substantive due process means that a disciplinary procedure must be fundamentally fair, especially in light of the fact that a health professional respondent faces potential loss of a constitutionally recognized property interest in the earned privilege of professional practice.

For disciplinary actions taken by voluntary, private (nongovernmental) associations and boards, constitutional due process considerations do not strictly apply.

As with news about other public figures, the public has the constitutional "right to know" about disciplinary actions taken by states against licensed or otherwise regulated health care professionals.

Instead, the internal affairs of voluntary private associations are governed by their own charters, constitutions, and bylaws. The private association analog of the requirement for due process is that these private associations must abide by their own rules and procedures when administering discipline.

Courts always have oversight jurisdiction over state administrative agencies and their decisions, as well as over the activities of voluntary, private associations. Courts are reluctant to reverse the decisions of governmental administrative agencies, however, for several reasons. These include deference to the reasonable decisions of administrative entities and considerations of time management. Reasons justifying reversal of administrative decisions include, for public agencies, the denial of due process to a respondent facing the loss of property or liberty interest, such as licensure to practice in a health care profession, and instances in which decisions are characterized as arbitrary, capricious, or the result of bias. Reasons for reversal of decisions of voluntary private associations include, among others, fraud, malice, bias, prejudicial failure to follow association rules and procedures, and instances in which decisions contravene law or public policy.

Summary

Health professional codes of ethics, similar to professional ethics codes in general, must be directive, protective of the public, specific to problems affecting a particular professional discipline, enforceable, and actually enforced. The rehabilitation professions all have governing codes of ethics with variable jurisdiction over practitioners in the specific disciplines.

Provisions within a given code of ethics are most commonly directive in nature but may be also nondirective, allowing for a greater exercise of individual judgment by practitioners. Disciplinary procedures for the professions of occupational therapy, orthotics and prosthetics, and physical therapy are similar, with minor variations, particularly regarding the reporting of disciplinary findings and sanctions.

> Private associations must abide by their own rules and procedures when administering discipline.

Cases and Questions

1. Using the illustrative health professional codes of ethics from this chapter and your own ethical standards and expectations, develop a comprehensive model interdisciplinary rehabilitation professional code of ethics.

2. A licensed rehabilitation health care professional is charged with intentional misconduct involving alleged sexual battery of a patient. In which venues might administrative or legal action take place, and what standards of proof apply to each action in each venue?

Suggested Answers for Cases and Questions

1. This project should be undertaken as a group exercise. After analysis of the representative codes of ethics and inclusion of the "best" provisions of each into the outline of the model code, the group should brainstorm over which additional provisions should be added to the model code.

2. A licensed rehabilitation health care professional charged with intentional misconduct involving a patient may face administrative and/or legal action in the following venues (applicable standards of proof appear in parentheses):

   a. Civil court for health care malpractice (preponderance, or greater weight, of evidence)
   b. Criminal court for felonious sexual battery (proof beyond a reasonable doubt)
   c. State licensure board (preponderance, or greater weight, of evidence)
   d. Professional association for unethical conduct (preponderance, or greater weight, of evidence)
   e. Certification entity for unethical conduct (preponderance, or greater weight, of evidence).

References

1. Richardson ML, White KK: *Ethics applied,* New York, 1993, McGraw-Hill, p 695.

2. American Physical Therapy Association: *Code of ethics and guide for professional conduct,* Alexandria, Va, 1997, APTA Judicial Committee, Section 1.1.

3. *Ibid.* Section 5.2C.

4. *Ibid.* Section 8.1.

5. American Board for Certification in Orthotics and Prosthetics: *Canons of ethical conduct,* Alexandria, Va, 1994, ABC Canon 2.1.

6. *Ibid.* Canon 3.2.

7. *Ibid.* Canon 2.5.

8. *Ibid.* Canon 6.1

9. American Physical Therapy Association: *Commonalities and differences between the professions of physical therapy and occupational therapy: an American physical therapy association white paper,* Alexandria, Va, 1995, APTA, p 32.

10. American Physical Therapy Association: *Procedural document on disciplinary action of the American physical therapy association,* Alexandria, Va, 1997, APTA.

11. American Physical Therapy Association: *Commonalities and differences between the professions of physical therapy and occupational therapy: an American physical therapy association white paper,* Alexandria, Va, 1995, APTA, p 34.

12. American Occupational Therapy Association: *Enforcement procedure for occupational therapy code of ethics,* Bethesda, Md, 1998, AOTA, as amended.

13. National Board for Certification in Occupational Therapy: *Press release: occupational therapy board announces new certification renewal program, changes name,* Gaithersburg, Md, 1996, NBCOT.

14. National Board for Certification in Occupational Therapy: *Procedures for disciplinary action,* Gaithersburg, Md, 1989, NBCOT.

15. Battle over OT designations might be resolved in court, *Nursing & Allied Healthweek* 4:8, (Apr. 7)1997.

16. American Board for Certification in Orthotics and Prosthetics: *Character and fitness rules and procedures: rules and procedures regarding ethical, character and fitness complaints,* Alexandria, Va, 1994, ABC, p 1.

17. *Ibid.* p 1.

18. In states in which unlicensed providers fall outside of the jurisdiction of state regulatory agencies, disciplinary action may be taken by the Office of the Attorney General. For more on this issue, see "Disciplinary procedures and unlicensed practitioners." *Federation of State Boards of Physical Therapy Newsletter* 11(10):2, 1996.

19. *Medical Boards of California Action Report,* Jan 1995, p 31.

20. Texas Board of Physical Therapy Examiners: Licensure suspension for nonpayment of child support, *Communique, Texas board of physical therapy examiners* (Fall) 1995, p 1..

21. Kyler P: *Everyday ethics: common concerns in occupational therapy,* Rockville, Md, 1995, AOTA, p 31.

22. American Board for Certification in Orthotics and Prosthetics: *Character and fitness rules and procedures: rules and procedures regarding ethical, character and fitness complaints,* Alexandria, Va, 1994, ABC, p 7.

23. Bennett JJ (General Counsel, APTA): *Memorandum* Oct 11, 1995, p 3.

Suggested Readings

American Board for Certification in Orthotics and Prosthetics: *Canons of ethical conduct,* Alexandria, Va, 1994, ABC.

American Board for Certification in Orthotics and Prosthetics: *Character and fitness rules and procedures: rules and procedures regarding ethical, character and fitness complaints,* Alexandria, Va, 1994, ABC.

American Nurses Association: *Code for nurses with interpretive statements,* Washington, DC, 1985, ANA.

American Occupational Therapy Association: *Enforcement procedure for occupational therapy code of ethics,* Bethesda, Md, 1998, AOTA, as amended.

American Occupational Therapy Association: *Occupational therapy code of ethics,* Bethesda, Md, 1994, AOTA Commission on Standards and Ethics.

American Physical Therapy Association: *Code of ethics and guide for professional conduct,* Alexandria, Va, 1997, APTA Judicial Committee.

American Physical Therapy Association: *Commonalities and differences between the professions of physical therapy and occupational therapy: an American physical therapy association white paper,* Alexandria, Va, 1995, APTA.

American Physical Therapy Association: *Procedural document on disciplinary action of the American Physical Therapy Association,* Alexandria, Va, 1997, APTA.

American Physical Therapy Association: *Standards of ethical conduct and guide for conduct of the affiliate member,* Alexandria, Va, 1997, APTA Judicial Committee.

Faso DR: *The canons of ethical conduct,* Dallas, Tex, (Sep 14)1995, University of Texas Southwestern Medical Center.

Association of Rehabilitation Nurses: *Position statement: ethical issues,* Glenview, Ill, 1994, Association of Rehabilitation Nurses.

Battle over OT designations might be resolved in court, *Nursing & Allied Healthweek* 4:8, (Apr. 7)1997.

Kyler P: *Everyday ethics: common concerns in occupational therapy,* Rockville, Md, 1995, AOTA, p 31.

McLaughlin C: Rehab nurses: integral members of rehab team, *Advance for Physical Therapists* Nov 18, 1996, p 22.

National Board for Certification in Occupational Therapy: *Procedures for disciplinary action,* Gaithersburg, Md, 1989, NBCOT.

Pierce MF: Pharmacy techs create code of ethics, *Nursing & Allied Healthweek* Nov 18, 1996, p 9.

Richardson ML, White KK: *Ethics applied,* New York, 1993, McGraw-Hill.

Smith R: The American speech-language-hearing association, *Rehab Management* Feb/Mar 1995, p 15.

Informed Consent Issues

This chapter overviews the ethical considerations and legal issues associated with patient and research subject informed consent to intervention and research, respectively. The common disclosure elements for patient informed consent— diagnosis and evaluative findings, recommended intervention, material risks of harm or complication, goals of intervention, and reasonable alternatives— are discussed in detail. Informed consent ethical issues related to human subject research are explored. This chapter ends with the analysis of managed care informed consent issues, including employment "gag clauses" restricting provider-patient communications and nondisclosure of provider financial conflicts of interest.

●

Patient Informed Consent to Intervention

Patient informed consent to intervention is one of the most important mixed ethical and legal issues impacting health care professional clinical practice. Every health care clinician has the ethical duty and, in the overwhelming majority of cases, the legal duty to obtain patient or surrogate informed consent to health care interventions. This obligation is incumbent not only upon physicians and surgeons but also on all other licensed and certified health care professionals, especially rehabilitation professionals. Incidentally, the obligation to obtain patient informed consent applies irrespective of whether a nonphysician health care professional evaluates and treats a patient with, or without, physician or other-provider referral.

Ethical Duty to Obtain Patient Informed Consent

Every health care professional has an ethical and legal duty to obtain patient informed consent to evaluation and intervention.

The ethical obligation to universally obtain patient or surrogate informed consent to health care evaluation and treatment is founded on the foundational ethical principle of autonomy.[1] Making relevant disclosure of information about evaluation and treatment and involving the patient in health care decision making evidences respect for patient self-determination.

All competent adult patients have the right to control the health care treatment decision-making process under the foundational ethical principle of autonomy.[2] Patients not considered legally competent to make such decisions—those who are legally adjudicated as incompetent, and minors, in some cases—have the right to have a surrogate decision maker or other legal representative receive the same disclosure information that would be imparted to a competent patient and make decisions for them.

For many centuries, the foundational ethical principle of respect for patient autonomy was not the preeminent guiding ethical principle governing health care delivery. Rather, physicians and other primary health care professionals conformed their conduct to another foundational ethical principle, beneficence, under which the health care professionals make and execute professional judgments that they believe to be in patients' best interests but do not routinely involve patients in decision making regarding interventions to be employed.[3]

The history of the development of the law and ethics of patient informed consent demonstrates that, until very recently, health care professionals practiced their professions largely without involving their patients in treatment-related decision making. Many explanations—some seemingly reasonable—have been proffered by medical and other health professions to justify unilateral decision making regarding health care interventions. The ancient Greeks believed that to involve patients in medical decision making would impair patients' confidence in the ability of their health care providers to make professional judgments. By the Middle Ages, it was widely believed that the use of deception was necessary to ensure patient compliance with prescribed medical treatment that was deemed to be in the patient's best interests.[4] Modernly, there is legitimate concern among health care professionals that patients will not understand and will be confused by the myriad of complex pieces of information that must be imparted as part of informed consent disclosure. Finally, with streamlined managed heath care delivery, there is even a sense among some health care providers that routinely obtaining patient consent to treatment is just too time-consuming.

The customary health professional practice of not including patients as partners in health care decision making began to change in the early and mid-1900s. Several phenomena accelerated the rise in importance of respect for patient autonomy in health care decision making. First, courts began to mandate that health care professionals respect patient autonomy and impart "legally sufficient" disclosure to permit patients to make knowing, intelligent, voluntary, and unequivocal elections of recommended treatment. The advent of this trend in judicial activism is exemplified by the 1914 New York case, *Schloendorf v. Society of New York Hospital*,[5] which expanded intentional tort liability in battery of health care providers who failed to respect the right of patients to knowingly consent to treatment. In 1965 in *Natanson v. Kline*,[6] the Kansas Supreme Court also ruled that:

> The courts frequently state that the relationship between the physician and his patient is a fiduciary one, and therefore the physician has the obligation to make a full and frank disclosure to the patient of all pertinent facts related to his illness. We are here concerned with a case where the physician is charged with treating the patient without consent on the grounds that the patient was not fully informed of the nature of the treatment or its consequences, and therefore "consent" obtained was ineffective.

In another leading informed consent case in 1972, *Canterbury v. Spence*,[7] Judge Spotswood Robinson III of the United States Court of Appeals for the District of Columbia further refined the nature of the ethical duty owed by health care professionals toward their patients. He stated:

> The patient's reliance upon the physician is a trust of the kind which traditionally has exacted obligations beyond those associated with arms length transactions. [The patient's] dependence upon the physician for information affecting his well-being, in terms of contemplated treatment, is well-nigh abject....

Other twentieth century developments that furthered the recognition of patient autonomy over decision making and the need for patient informed consent in health care service delivery include the growth in postsecondary education after

The history of the development of the law and ethics of patient informed consent demonstrates that, until very recently, health care professionals practiced their professions largely without involving their patients in treatment-related decision making.

World War II and the concomitant rise of the consumerism movement in the United States and Canada and later in Western Europe. As consumers became more aware of their power over merchants in the retail industry, the age-old adage, *caveat emptor* (Latin for "let the buyer beware") became whittled away as the public forcefully lobbied federal and state legislators for the enactment of consumer protection laws. As a result of consumer protection legislation, the doctrine of *caveat emptor* largely came to have little meaning in retail consumer business transactions. About the same time, it was realized that this doctrine was even less appropriately applied in the delivery of health services to patients.

Many health professional association codes of ethics expressly recognize an ethical duty on the part of professional members to make sufficient disclosure of pertinent information to patients under their care to permit patients to make informed elections about treatment. For example, the Guide for Professional Conduct, governing ethical behavior for physical therapist members of the American Physical Therapy Association, states in pertinent part, "Physical therapists shall obtain patient informed consent before treatment."[8] Similarly, the Occupational Therapy Code of Ethics, governing the ethical conduct of occupational therapist members of the American Occupational Therapy Association, states in pertinent parts, "Occupational therapy personnel shall fully inform [patients] of the nature, risks, and potential outcomes of any intervention."[9] "Occupational therapy personnel shall respect the individual's right to refuse professional services or involvement in research or educational activities."[10]

Legal Aspects of Patient Informed Consent to Treatment

Failure to Obtain Patient Informed Consent Is a Form of Health Care Malpractice

Failure on the part of health care professionals to make necessary disclosure of evaluative and treatment-related information, so as to enable patients to make informed decisions about treatment options, constitutes professional negligence—the most common variety of health care malpractice. Until very recently, lack of informed consent tort cases in health care settings were treated as intentional tort actions and were processed through the civil legal system as battery cases.[11] The rationale for labeling lack of informed consent health care malpractice cases as battery cases was that physicians and other health care professionals charged with such malpractice actions were considered by law to have had harmful physical contact with their patients without such patients' consent. By 1965, when the *Natanson v. Kline*[12] decision was announced, courts began to realize that there was a fundamental distinction between consent-related cases that involved intentional wrongs (i.e., based on a lack of autho-

Failure of health care professionals to make necessary disclosure of evaluative and treatment-related information to patients constitutes professional negligence—the most common variety of health care malpractice.

rization) and those that involved unintentional wrongs (i.e., based on a lack of under-standing); the courts began to correctly classify lack of informed consent health care malpractice cases as professional negligence actions, since patients treated without informed consent probably would have given at least nominal (albeit uninformed) consent to the treatment that led to injury.

Certain consent-related actions still are properly brought as intentional battery cases. For example, when a surgeon operates on a patient and amputates the wrong limb, or excises the wrong breast or testicle during a mastectomy or orchiecto-my, respectively, or when a nurse administers the wrong medication to a patient, caus-ing patient injury, the proper designation for the ensuing legal action is a "battery." This is so because the defendant–health care professional involved had absolutely no authorization from the injured patient to carry out inappropriate and harmful treat-ment.

The professional negligence designation for lack of informed consent health care malpractice cases takes into account the fact that patients injured in such cases probably gave nominal consent to treatment, but their health care providers failed to conform with acceptable practice standards by neglecting to respect patient autonomy by involving the patients in treatment-related decision making. Therefore failure to obtain patient informed consent to treatment equates to substandard care—the essence of health care professional negligence.

Only one state's legal system, Pennsylvania, still considers lack of informed consent to be a battery.[15] As will be illustrated in the next section, Pennsylvania is also the only state whose state and federal courts have ruled that health care providers in nonoperative settings have no legal obligation under state law to obtain patient informed consent for health care interventions.

Failure to obtain patient-informed consent to treatment equates to substandard care.

Legal Recognition of the Obligation to Obtain Patient Informed Consent

Except under Pennsylvania law, the right of patients to give informed consent to health care interventions is clearly recognized as a fundamental legal right, by statute, case law, and/or customary professional health care practice, in every jurisdiction in the United States. This legal obligation is reflected in health professional written practice standards, such as those of the American Physical Therapy Association[14] and of other rehabilitation professions.

The Pennsylvania courts have ruled on at least two occasions that informed consent in the health care setting is a concept reserved exclusively for surgi-cal and operative procedures—not for routine health care delivery.[15,16] In *Spence v. Todaro,* the Federal District Court for the Eastern District of Pennsylvania, interpret-ing Pennsylvania state law, specifically held that the doctrine of informed consent to treatment does not apply to postoperative physical therapy rehabilitation. This case concerned a postoperative orthopedic patient who was referred to physical therapy for rotator cuff rehabilitation. The patient claimed injury incident to physical therapy and sued the physical therapist for malpractice, citing a lack of informed consent as the basis for his lawsuit. The federal court held that, under Pennsylvania statutory law, the doctrine of patient informed consent to treatment applies only to surgical interventions—not to routine (nonsurgical) health care delivery. The court went on to reject the plaintiff-patient's contention that, because his physical therapy followed directly from his rotator cuff repair, it was legally part of the surgery, thereby making his lack of informed consent a valid issue for judicial review.

In all other health care legal cases, however, the doctrine of patient informed consent to treatment has been found applicable, either expressly or by implication, to nonsurgical cases and to nonphysician primary health care providers. For example, in *Flores v. Center for Spinal Evaluation*,[17] a physical and occupational therapy malpractice case involving an allegation of professional negligence incident to postinjury rehabilitation, the court held in dismissing the case that, despite limited legal precedent on physical and occupational therapy malpractice, these health care professionals (and by analogy, other rehabilitation professionals) should be treated exactly like their physician colleagues when they are health care malpractice defendants.

Recent United States Supreme Court case decisions interpreting the Constitution have reflected the Court's deference to and respect for patient self-determination regarding important health care decision making. For example, United States Supreme Court case decisions (and those of state supreme and appellate courts) based on the fundamental right of privacy have favored patients in their decisions to compel removal of life support apparatus[18] and even the withdrawal of nutrition and hydration.[19,20]

In many states, including Florida, Georgia, Idaho, Iowa, Louisiana, Maine, Nevada, North Carolina, Ohio, Texas, Utah, and West Virginia, state legislatures have enacted statutes that mandate the specific informed consent disclosure required for surgical procedures and anesthesia administration, as a matter of law. In these states, compliance with statutory disclosure, coupled with the signature of a patient on a statutory form, creates a rebuttable presumption that the patient gave informed consent to care. The burden of persuasion to dispute or rebut that presumption in litigation then shifts to the patient.

Another (federal) statute, the Patient Self-Determination Act[21] (discussed in greater detail in Chapter 8), codifies the rights of hospitalized inpatients and nursing home residents to participate in treatment decision making and to control the use of extraordinary treatment measures, such as artificial life support. The Patient Self-Determination Act, although not creating any new substantive legal requirements for health care organizations or rights for patients, binds all health care facilities that receive Medicare or Medicaid funding to inform patients about their existing substantive rights under state law and to respect legitimate patients' advance directives concerning treatment. Regarding informed consent, the law provides in pertinent part[22] that:

> [A] provider [must] maintain written policies and procedures with respect to all adult individuals receiving medical care...to provide written information to each such individual concerning an individual's rights under state law (whether statutory or as recognized by the courts of the state) to make decisions concerning...medical care, including the right to accept or refuse medical or surgical treatment.

Another source of legal obligation to obtain patient informed consent is the American Hospital Association's Patient Bill of Rights,[23] a document customarily posted in patient treatment areas in health care facilities across the United States. The Patient Bill of Rights states in pertinent part:

> We consider you a partner in your hospital care. When you are well-informed, participate in treatment decisions, and communicate openly with your doctor and other health professionals, you help make your care as effective as possible. This hospital encourages respect for the personal preferences and values of each individual.
>
> While you are a patient in the hospital, your rights include the following:
>
> You have the right to be well-informed about your illness, possible treatments, and likely outcome and to discuss this information with your doctor. You have the right to know the names and roles of people treating you.
>
> You have the right to consent to or refuse a treatment, as permitted by law, throughout your hospital stay. If you refuse a recommended treatment, you will [still] receive other needed and available care.
>
> You have the right to have an advance directive, such as a living will or health care proxy. These documents express your choices about your future care or name someone to decide if you cannot speak for yourself. If you have a written advance directive, you should provide a copy to the hospital, your family, and your doctor.
>
> If transfer is recommended or requested, you will be informed of risks, benefits, and alternatives.
>
> You have the right to know if this hospital has relationships with outside parties that may influence your treatment and care. These relationships may be with educational institutions, other health care providers, or insurers.
>
> You have the right to consent or decline to take part in research affecting your care. If you choose not to take part, you will [still] receive the most effective care the hospital otherwise provides.
>
> You have the right to be told of realistic care alternatives when hospital care is no longer appropriate.

51

You have the right to know about hospital rules that affect you and your treatment and about charges and payment methods. You have the right to know about hospital resources, such as patient representatives or ethics committees, that can help you resolve problems and questions about your hospital stay and care.

In carrying out these activities, this institution works to respect your values and dignity.

The Joint Commission on the Accreditation of Health Care Organizations (JCAHO), like other private accreditation entities, imposes similar requirements on its member health care organizations. Specifically, JCAHO standards require appropriate evidence in patient health records of informed consent to treatment, as well as institutional policy statements on patient informed consent.[24]

Finally, health care organizations and networks can create legally binding standards regarding patient informed consent in their organizational procedures manuals, protocols, and clinical practice guidelines, over and above those otherwise required by law. Administrators and clinical managers are urged to review these types of documents to ensure that what is written therein reflects what is desired practice standards for the organization.

When Is Lack of Patient Informed Consent Legally Actionable?

Even though every single unexcused and unjustified omission of patient informed consent is an example of professional negligence, only a limited number of instances are legally actionable. Professional negligence malpractice litigation premised on a lack of informed consent is legally actionable only when:

- an undisclosed risk materializes, resulting in patient injury; and
- the plaintiff-patient can establish (i.e., prove) that he or she would not have consented to the treatment intervention in issue had full disclosure been made.

The court in *Canterbury*[25] clearly spells out the requirement for a causal connection between the negligent omission on the part of a health care clinician to make legally sufficient disclosure to a patient and resultant patient injury.

No more than breach of any other legal duty does nonfulfillment of the physician's obligation to disclose alone establish liability to the patient. *An unrevealed risk that should have been made known must materialize, for otherwise the omission, however unpardonable, is legally without consequence. Occurrence of the risk must be harmful to the patient, for unrelated to injury is nonactionable* [emphasis added]. And, as in malpractice actions generally,

Rehabilitation professionals are strongly advised to universally make the informed disclosure and patient consent process an integral part of their patient evaluation and intervention processes.

there must be a causal relationship between the physician's failure to adequately divulge (information) and damage to the patient.

A causal connection exists when, but only when, disclosure of significant risks incidental to treatment would have resulted in a decision against it [emphasis added]. The patient obviously has no complaint if he would have submitted to the therapy notwithstanding awareness that the risk was one of its perils. On the other hand, the very purpose of the disclosure rule is to protect the patient against the consequences which, if known, he would have avoided by foregoing the treatment.

Litigation over informed consent to treatment should never occur if health care professionals remember that disclosure of treatment-related information is a requisite element of the provider-patient communication process. The disclosure elements (discussed below) are relatively straightforward, and the process, if made a routine part of provider-patient communications, is neither unduly burdensome nor time-consuming.

Obviously, open and thorough communication between health care providers and patients is key to minimizing health care malpractice liability exposure. The word "consent" literally means that the provider and patient jointly should agree on a recommended treatment intervention before it is implemented.[26] Decades of medical research have shown that patients achieve optimal intervention outcomes when they are informed partners in their own care.[27]

One confounding factor to the health care provider–patient communication process is the fact that some patients, especially geriatric patients, may wish not to participate in the treatment decision-making process with their providers. Rather, some patients—even though they are fully competent to do so—prefer to leave treatment decision making to family members or trusted others. Regarding revelation of terminal illnesses, this impediment to provider-patient communications may be race- or ethnicity-related. One study revealed that, whereas African and white geriatric Americans generally believe that it is appropriate for providers to discuss terminal illnesses with their patients, Korean and Mexican-Americans often do not.[28] In complicated fact scenarios like those presented in this exemplar, health care clinicians are strongly encouraged to consult with facility and/or personal legal advisors for advice on how to proceed and to carefully document their actions.

Disclosure Elements for Legally Sufficient Disclosure of Information to Patients

Although legal requirements differ from state to state for what constitutes legally sufficient information disclosure in the provider-patient informed consent communication process, the following elements are commonly included in most or all states. For spe-

Disclosure of information to patients is relatively straightforward, and the process, if made a routine part of provider-patient communications, is neither unduly burdensome nor time-consuming.

cific advice on what information must be imparted to patients under a specific state's laws, consult with legal counsel.

For patient consent to treatment to be legally "informed," the following items of disclosure information should be addressed:

● *Diagnosis and pertinent evaluative findings.* Health care clinicians should always discuss with patients the patients' diagnoses and pertinent evaluative findings (unless the patient effectively waives disclosure or another exception applies). Although it may be particularly difficult for health care professionals to avoid the use of health professional jargon in communications because of their training, communication with other providers, and continuing education, they must remember to speak to patients using layperson's language and at a level of understanding appropriate for each patient.

● *Nature of the treatment intervention recommended.* After patient evaluation is completed and a diagnosis is made, a clinician formulates a proposed treatment plan designed to optimize function or achieve some other therapeutic result. This recommended treatment intervention must be disclosed to the patient before its implementation, and the patient must agree to treatment. If specific treatment has been prescribed by a physician or other provider legally privileged to make referrals, then the prescribed treatment must likewise be described to the patient. In either case, the patient must consent to treatment.

● *Material (decisional) risks of serious harm or complications.* Any credible risk of possible serious harm or complication associated with a proposed treatment intervention must be disclosed to a patient before treatment commences. The term *material* refers to a risk of harm that would cause an ordinary reasonable patient to think seriously about whether he or she would accept or reject a proposed treatment intervention. (In some cases, the term *material* has been construed by courts to mean the risk of harm that a particular patient would subjectively consider to be serious, even if that particular patient was not an ordinary reasonable person.) It is often said that there are few material risks of serious harm or complications associated with physical and occupational therapy and orthotic and prosthetic interventions. This is probably true; however, there are a number of discipline-specific material risks that must be disclosed to patients. One nonobvious material risk associated with physical therapy involves axillary crutch gait instruction. Unless a physical therapist warns a patient about the material risk of possible axillary nerve and vessel injury associated with leaning on the soft axillary pads on the top portions of the crutches, a patient might reasonably believe that the soft pads are designed to be leaned upon. By disclosing this potential risk, a physical therapist may prevent patient injury and malpractice litigation. Another material risk of harm that must be disclosed—by prosthetists providing artificial limbs to clients—is the risk of harm associated with skin breakdown around a pros-

Recommended treatment intervention must be described to the patient before its implementation, and the patient must agree to the treatment.

thesis. A patient must be informed by his or her prosthetist that the signs and symptoms of pain, redness, and skin breakdown in the vicinity of a prosthesis are not normal and may result in serious adverse consequences and must immediately be made known by the patient to his or her providers. The law generally recognizes that the only material risks that need to be disclosed to patients are those that are nonobvious to ordinary reasonable people. Obvious risks, such as the risk of being cut by a sharp needle or of being burned by an extremely hot thermal treatment modality, are generally understood by adult lay patients and are not required to be discussed. However, patients may not fully comprehend the gravity of the risk of harm associated with seemingly obvious risk scenarios. Consider the following hypothetical example:

A 68-year-old male patient with a medical diagnosis of diabetes mellitus and a left lateral malleolar diabetic ulcer on his ankle is referred to physical therapy for "evaluation and hydrotherapy, as appropriate." After evaluation and initial treatment, the physical therapist advises the patient to soak his left foot in very warm water at home for 20 minutes, twice a day. The patient asks, "How warm should the water be?" The therapist replies, "As warm as you can tolerate on the unaffected part of your left foot." Unfortunately, the physical therapist had neglected to evaluate the patient's whole foot, which was severely desensitized as a result of peripheral neuropathy. The next day, the patient returns to the clinic with third-degree thermal burns to his left foot. The patient had boiled water, poured it into a basin, and placed his left foot into the scalding water, resulting in serious injury. The patient's left foot was amputated several weeks later.

Out of concern for patient welfare and as a matter of prudent risk management, the health care provider should always discuss even seemingly obvious risks of serious harm or complications of treatment with patients to prevent needless patient injury and liability exposure.

● *Expected benefits of treatment.* It is incumbent upon health care clinicians to establish functionally relevant, measurable, short- and long-term treatment goals for patients under their care. As an integral part of the informed consent process, health care clinicians must also reveal and discuss with patients the goals established for them. If patients understand the treatment goals established on their behalf and take an "ownership" interest in the treatment goals, they will be more motivated to achieve better functional outcomes.

● *Reasonable alternatives to the proposed intervention.* If there are reasonable alternatives to a proposed treatment or intervention, these must be dis-

If patients understand the treatment goals established on their behalf and take an "ownership" interest in the treatment goals, they will be more motivated to achieve better functional outcomes.

55

closed to and discussed with the patient. In addition to describing reasonable alternatives to proposed treatments, clinicians must also discuss with patients the attendant material risks (if any) and expected benefits of such reasonable alternatives. This disclosure element may pose a problem under managed care, in that alternative treatments or interventions, even if more efficacious than a recommended treatment, may not be available or funded under the patient's managed care plan. This fact does not, however, obviate the need for discussion of all reasonable alternative treatments or interventions.

After disclosing all informed consent parameters to a patient—diagnostic and evaluative findings, nature of recommended treatment, material risks, expected benefits, and reasonable alternatives (Box 3-1)—a health care clinician is obliged to take one further step. The provider must ensure that the patient understands all the information conveyed by asking for and by satisfactorily answering patient questions related to treatment. If the patient's primary language is one other than English, the provider must provide translation, as needed, to ensure that all information conveyed is understood by the patient.

Box 3-1. Informed Consent to Treatment

Disclosure of relevant treatment-related information includes:

Patient diagnosis or evaluative findings

Nature of treatment or intervention recommended or ordered

Material (decisional) risks of serious harm or complication associated with the proposed treatment or intervention

Expected benefits or goals associated with the proposed treatment or intervention

Reasonable alternatives, if any, to the proposed treatment or intervention

---

Occasionally, a patient will refuse treatment recommended by a health care provider or ordered by a physician or other referring entity, even after informed consent disclosure has been made. Certain additional steps must be taken by a health care provider whenever a patient refuses care. The clinician must first ensure that the patient understands the disclosure information conveyed and must solicit further questions or comments about the proposed treatment or intervention that the patient may have to offer. If this reiteration and summarization of the informed consent process does not resolve the problem, the clinician should explain, in an empathetic and objective manner, the expected consequences of refusal of treatment or intervention to the patient's health status, as applicable. Discussion with the patient should be interactive and participative rather than directive, and the clinician should display both sincere concern for the patient's best health interests (beneficence) and respect for patient autonomy over decision making.

If the patient persists in his or her refusal to allow recommended treatment, this fact and a summarization of the "informed refusal" prevention measures employed on the patient's behalf should be well documented in the patient's health record. In addition, the clinician is legally and ethically responsible to coordinate expeditiously with the referring entity, if any, and other key health care professionals having a need to know about the patient's refusal of care.

Legal Standards for Adequacy of Informed Consent

There are two possible legal standards used to determine whether a health care professional made sufficient disclosure of treatment-related information in order to permit a patient to make an informed decision about care. The states are nearly equally divided in their use of each available standard; however, a slight majority of jurisdictions use a *professional standard* for disclosure.[29] In states employing this legal disclosure standard, a health care professional is required to impart to a patient only that information that another health professional from the same discipline, who would be acting under the same or similar circumstances, would see fit to disclose. Health care malpractice litigation involving informed consent issues in states using the professional standard requires the introduction of expert testimony concerning: (1) the propriety of the disclosure information actually conveyed by a defendant–health care provider to a plaintiff-patient, and (2) the expert's professional opinion about what information is generally appropriate for disclosure to patients under the same or similar circumstances.

A slight minority of states employ a *layperson's standard* for disclosure. In these jurisdictions, a health care professional is required to disclose all relevant information that an ordinary reasonable patient, acting under the same or similar circumstances as the patient in issue, would consider *material* to make an informed decision about treatment. Obviously, the lay standard imposes greater responsibility on health care providers, who must carefully contemplate what information an ordinary reasonable lay patient would deem to be *material* for every possible treatment or intervention.

The court in *Canterbury* enunciated in a very reasoned manner the rationale for and the parameters of the ordinary reasonable layperson's standard for the first time as follows:

> We do not agree that the patient's cause of action is dependent upon the existence and nonperformance of a relevant professional tradition. There are, in our view, formidable obstacles to acceptance of the notion that [a health care professional's] obligation to disclose is either germinated or lim-

If a patient refuses treatment, this fact and a summarization of the "informed refusal" prevention measures employed on the patient's behalf should be well-documented...the clinician is legally and ethically responsible to coordinate with any referring health care professional about the patient's refusal of care.

ited by medical practice. To begin with, the reality of any discernible custom reflecting a professional consensus on communication of option and risk information to patients is open to serious doubt. We sense the danger that what in fact is no custom at all may be taken as an affirmative custom to maintain silence, and that [health professional–witnesses] to the so-called custom may state merely their personal opinions as to what they or others would do under given conditions.

The decision to unveil the patient's condition and the chances for as to remediation...is ofttimes a non-medical judgment and, if so, is a decision outside the ambit of the special standard....Prevailing medical practice...does not...define the standard.

In our view, the patient's right of self-decision shapes the boundaries of the duty to reveal. That right can be effectively exercised only if the patient possesses enough information to enable an intelligent choice. The scope of the [provider's] communication to the patient, then, must be measured by the patient's need, and that need is the information *material* [emphasis added] to the decision. Thus the test for determining whether a particular peril must be divulged is its materiality to the [ordinary reasonable] patient's decision: all risks potentially affecting the decision must be unmasked.

One advantage to both parties to an informed consent-based health care malpractice lawsuit of the application by the court of the layperson standard for assessing disclosure is that, under most circumstances, expert testimony about health professional discipline-specific disclosure standards is not required, since it is the responsibility of lay jurors to decide what information an ordinary reasonable patient would need to hear in order to make an informed decision about accepting or rejecting treatment. This fact saves money at trial that otherwise would be paid to expert witnesses, which benefits both parties to the lawsuit. Additionally, when expert witnesses are not utilized in a case, substantial time is usually saved in litigating the material issues in the case.

Exceptions to the Requirement to Obtain Patient Informed Consent

There are several well-established exceptions to the requirement to otherwise universally obtain patient informed consent before carrying out health care treatment interventions. The two most important ones are the *emergency doctrine* and *therapeutic privilege.*[30]

Under the emergency doctrine, whenever a patient seeks evaluation and treatment in a life-threatening emergency situation and is unable to communicate his or her wishes regarding treatment (such as when the patient is unconscious), it is generally presumed that the patient would consent to reasonable, life-saving medical intervention. Consider the following hypothetical case scenario.

> A student orthotist in a clinical affiliation is evaluating a 65-year-old male rehabilitation patient, who is recovering from a left cerebrovascular accident, for the fitting of a spiral right lower limb orthosis. Suddenly, the patient suffers a myocardial infarction and grasps his chest. The patient is initially unable to speak because of pain and shortness of breath; he then becomes unconscious. What action should the student take? (At the time of the incident, there is no one, including the student's supervisory clinical instructor, in the clinic area.)

This scenario presents an example of a situation in which the emergency doctrine exception to the law of patient informed consent is applicable. In such a situation, it is generally presumed, as a matter of law, that an ordinary reasonable person would wish to avail himself or herself of life-saving treatment intervention. Absent clear evidence of contrary patient desires, the student should immediately commence cardiopulmonary resuscitation and activate the emergency medical response system.

There are, of course, exceptions to the exception of a presumption favoring rendition of care in life-threatening emergencies. For example, if a patient's desire not to receive life-saving care in the event of an emergency has been memorialized in a valid patient advance directive (discussed in detail in Chapter 8), health care professionals and supportive personnel are obligated to respect the patient's autonomy and not initiate life-saving treatment. A similar exception applies when a valid "do not resuscitate" order appears in a patient's medical record.

Do not resuscitate (DNR) orders preclude the otherwise automatic initiation of cardiopulmonary resuscitation efforts for a patient in cardiorespiratory arrest. A DNR order does *not* affect the provision of any other substantive care, such as life support and nutrition and hydration. A DNR order may be appropriate either to respect the prior choice of a patient regarding treatment or when, in the professional judgment of a patient's attending physician (normally with the concurrence of at least one other physician), resuscitative efforts for a patient would be medically futile. DNR orders are written for patients who are terminally ill or living in a persistent vegetative state.[31] Because of complex legal and ethical issues surrounding DNR orders and other decisions involving life support and nutrition and hydration of patients, health care professionals confronting these situations are urged to expeditiously consult with facility legal counsel and institutional ethics committees for advice. Clinical managers should involve legal counsel and bioethicists and applied ethicists in inservice educa-

If a patient's desire not to receive life-saving care in the event of an emergency has been memorialized in a valid patient advance directive, health care professionals and supportive personnel are obligated to respect the patient's autonomy and not initiate life-saving treatment.

tional experiences with clinical staff caring for patients for whom DNR orders are or might be written.

Therapeutic privilege is the other major exception to informed consent law.[32] Under therapeutic privilege, a physician may be legally and ethically justified in withholding in good faith information from a patient about his or her diagnosis or prognosis when, in the physician's professional judgment, the patient cannot deal psychologically with the information. The exercise of a therapeutic privilege by a physician to withhold diagnostic or prognostic information from a patient does not excuse the physician (or other health care professionals treating the patient) from disclosing any other pertinent information to the patient.

Therapeutic privilege is rarely invoked and even less often sanctioned by the courts as legally acceptable. This is so because the exercise of the privilege derogates from the foundational biomedical ethical principle of respect for patient autonomy and self-determination.

What course of action can a nonphysician health care professional treating a patient take when he or she disagrees with a physician's invocation of therapeutic privilege? Consider the following hypothetical case example:

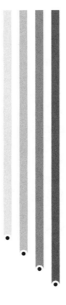

An occupational therapist treating a 32-year-old female patient, who is diagnosed with terminal, end-stage metastatic breast cancer, meets with the other rehabilitation team members for a weekly team conference. At the meeting, the patient's attending physician advises the team members that he is discharging the patient to home to allow her to die in peace with her family. The attending physician tells the team treating the patient that he is invoking therapeutic privilege concerning the patient's prognosis. (The patient already knows her diagnosis.) The occupational therapist knows, from her recent conversations with the patient, that the patient wishes to know about her prognosis and apprises the rest of the team of this fact. The physician becomes angry and reminds the occupational therapist that he is the patient's physician and the leader of the rehabilitation team. The physician ends the discussion by imposing a "gag order" on the entire treatment team, ordering all of them to remain silent if asked by the patient about her prognosis.

Is this the end of the matter? Not necessarily. In this case, the occupational therapist is unable to abide by the physician's decision as a matter of personal ethics. What can she do? There are several acceptable options open to the occupational therapist. First, the occupational therapist should consider requesting a private meeting with the physician to express her concerns about the gag order. Assume that she does this and poignantly states her position. Assume further that her resistance to his edict enrages the physician, who summarily ejects the occupational therapist from his office stating, "Just do what I ordered!"

At this point, there are three options open to the occupational therapist. She may either resign herself to acceptance of the physician's order. However, in this case the patient, who has become accustomed to confiding in the occupational therapist, begins to pressure her for information about her prognosis. Additionally, the occupational therapist's personal code of ethics will not allow her to be untruthful to the patient.

The occupational therapist may, at this point, be justified in removing herself from the patient's treatment team—since she cannot abide by the physician's order—and allowing another occupational therapist who can accept the "gag order" to continue to care for the patient. However, in this case, the occupational therapist believes that this option is unethical and therefore an unacceptable "cop-out."

The last available option to the occupational therapist is perhaps the best one, after exercising all reasonable efforts to discuss the situation civilly with the physician. This option is to formally request an ethics consultation from the *institutional ethics committee* in the facility. The institutional ethics committee is a multidisciplinary committee of health care professionals and other related professionals that offers consultative services and convenes to hear and make recommendations about cases involving ethical dilemmas (among other roles; see Chapter 9). There should always be in place in any health care organization a mechanism for licensed and certified health care professionals and others to avail themselves of the advice and intervention of the institutional ethics committee. There should also never be any stigma associated with requesting consultation from the institutional ethics committee. Similarly, the fact that the occupational therapist acted reasonably in requesting an ethics consultation should not cause her to suffer retribution from the physician whose judgment is challenged. It may be necessary for facility administrators to educate physicians and other health professionals about the role(s) of the institutional ethics committee on a regular basis, so that misunderstandings and anger over its intervention do not occur.

Two other scenarios (involving the treatment of incompetent or minor patients) may seem to be possible exceptions to the requirement to obtain patient informed consent to treatment; however, such is not the case. When a patient is legally incompetent to consent to treatment—either because the patient cannot understand information conveyed and is a legally adjudicated incompetent, or because the patient is a minor and cannot consent to a particular intervention as a matter of law—a health care professional must obtain informed consent from a *surrogate* (or substitute) *decision maker.*

Therapeutic privilege is rarely invoked and even less often sanctioned by the courts as legally acceptable, because the privilege derogates from the foundational biomedical ethical principle of respect for patient autonomy and self-determination.

The disclosure of information made to a surrogate decision maker is exactly the same as would be made to a competent patient. The surrogate decision maker, appointed either by the patient or by law, acts on the patient's behalf and has the same right to have key information disclosed and to have questions answered to the surrogate's satisfaction, before treatment commences.

One exception to the general rule that parents or guardians normally consent on behalf of their minor children is that minors, especially when they are nearing the age of majority (age 18), may have the right under applicable state law to exercise autonomy to personally consent (usually without revelation to their parents) to treatment in cases involving elective abortion, treatment of drug (including alcohol) abuse, and the treatment of sexually transmitted diseases. These exceptions to the general rule of substituted consent for minors vary from state to state, and providers must consult proactively with legal counsel to remain current on the state of the law, so as to protect the rights of all parties.

Another difficult dilemma involving incompetent patients centers around informed consent involving patients who, practically but not legally, are incompetent to make knowing, intelligent, voluntary, and unequivocal decisions about treatment. Although the determination of patient competency to make decisions about health care interventions is a question for physicians and jurists, other health care professionals involved in the care of particular patients can offer important input into competency decisions, based on their observations and interactions with patients.

There is relatively little guidance in the health professional literature for physicians and other health care professionals on mental competency assessment. One excellent article on the topic that presents a framework for patient competency assessment (including dimensions of competence and a series of questions to assess mental capacity) is "Assessing Patient Competence for Medical Decision Making."[33] In cases of questionable patient competency to make treatment-related decisions, health care professionals are urged to raise the issue expeditiously with physicians, facility administrators, legal counsel, and institutional ethics committees, so that a competency determination can be undertaken, if appropriate. When a question of patient competency exists, a competency assessment is required to comply with legal requirements concerning consent to care and to meet foundational ethical standards, including respect for patient autonomy and dignity, beneficence, and nonmaleficence.

Informed Consent Issues in Research Settings

The informed consent of human research subjects is a fundamental requirement of and prerequisite to carrying out clinical research involving people. The process of

> The informed consent of human research subjects is a fundamental requirement of and prerequisite to carrying out clinical research involving people.

obtaining research subject informed consent is more complex than for obtaining patient informed consent to routine health care interventions. In part, this is because research-related consent is subject to greater institutional, administrative, and legal oversight than treatment-related informed consent, and in part because research-related subject consent normally must be documented in long-form, according to strict, rather than flexible, standards. (Documentation standards for patient informed consent to treatment or related intervention are more varied; individual documentation in patient health records of treatment-related informed consent may not even be ethically and legally required.[34])

The intense regulation of human subject research resulted in large part from the Nuremberg trials that followed World War II. In those trials, approximately twenty prominent German physicians were tried for human rights violations involving cruel and inhumane medical experimentation of prisoners of war. Most were convicted, and several were hanged.

Subsequent to the Nuremberg trials, the Nuremberg Code of 1947 was drafted and adopted. This code, in part, established as codified international law that "the voluntary consent of the human subject is absolutely essential" (to legally and ethically carry out permissible medical research).[35] The Nuremberg Code was augmented in 1975 by the Helsinki Declarations of 1964 (I) and 1975 (II), which established the international law requirement of independent review of research proposals involving human subjects as follows: "The design and performance of each experimental procedure involving human subjects should be clearly formulated in an experimental protocol which should be transmitted to a specially appointed independent committee for consideration, comment, and guidance."[36]

Based in large part on these international treaties and on human rights abuses in the American Tuskegee Syphilis Study, the Department of Health and Human Services (then the Department of Health, Education, and Welfare) adopted human subject research guidelines in the late 1970s that delineated the permissible scope of and procedures for human subject research activities that use federal funding. These guidelines also established the requirement for independent review of human subject research protocols by institutional review boards (IRBs). The federal guidelines were amended in 1981 to delete the requirement for IRB approval of a limited class of very low risk human subject research protocols.[37]

There are special federal guidelines regarding required elements that must be included in human subject research informed consent forms. These guidelines include the following parameters:

• The consent form must impart sufficient information about a proposed study, its procedures, expected benefits, material risks, and reasonable alternatives to enable a potential subject to make a knowing, intelligent, and voluntary decision about whether to agree to participate.

● The investigator (or approved designee) must personally explain the parameters to the potential subject.

● The consent form must be written in the first person, and must be in layperson's language, without significant technical medical "jargon." If the potential subject's language of comprehension is other than English, a translation of the consent form is required.

● In general, consent forms from other institutions may not be used to obtain human subject research consent.

● The consequences of subject injury must be clearly spelled out, including therapeutic measures to be taken in the event of subject injury and who bears the cost of such care.

● Any compensation or benefit that the subject will receive for participation in a research study must be clearly stated in the informed consent form.

● A copy of the signed form must be given to the subject. If the subject is also a patient, a copy of the research consent form must be filed in the patient's medical treatment record. The original copy of the consent form must be retained for at least 5 years after completion of the study.

● The consent form must be witnessed. The witness or witnesses attest only to a subject's signature, not to the subject's comprehension of disclosure elements or comprehension of them.

● The informed consent form must state contact telephone numbers for the principal investigator, where the subject can personally reach the investigator 24 hours a day.

Additional safeguards for research subject protection include:

● No person may be excluded from consideration as a research subject because of race, ethnicity, or language. The equitable inclusion of women and minorities in research is strongly encouraged.

● The subject's confidentiality and autonomy enjoy absolute respect and protection. The subject has the right to review all data collected from and about him or her and to withhold permission for their use by the researcher.

● The subject may withdraw consent at any time, without prejudice.

● The subject may not be prejudiced in receiving necessary and equitable care based on a decision not to participate in a research study.

Judicial activism is strong in protecting the rights of medical research subjects. In a recent case, *T.D. v. New York Office of Mental Health*,[38] the court ruled that nontherapeutic research involving greater than minimal risk of harm to minors and incompetent adult subjects is illegal under New York state law, based on the fact that these subjects cannot give informed consent to participate. In so ruling, New York became the eleventh state to ban such research. (The same rule of law applies in the United Kingdom.[39])

Patient Informed Consent in an Era of Managed Care

The managed care model of health care delivery has spawned at least two informed consent–related ethical dilemmas for health care professionals. First, compliance by providers with "gag clauses" in health professional employment contracts with managed care organizations may result in situations in which clinicians do not make full disclosure of treatment-related information to patients. Second, nondisclosure by health care professionals to patients of financial incentives paid to them for providing less care to patients fails to respect patient autonomy over treatment-related decision making.

"Gag clauses" are provisions in health professional–managed care organization employment contracts that obstruct a provider's ability to make full disclosure to patients of treatment-related information.[40] When a health care professional chooses to comply with a managed care "gag clause" provision and thereby places his or her own employment interests above patient welfare considerations, nondisclosure of key treatment-related information during informed consent processes may result. In particular, compliance by health care professionals with managed care "gag clauses" may prevent patients from receiving information about reasonable alternatives to proposed interventions not funded by patients' insurance plans. Many managed care plans have backed away from "gag clauses" in employment contracts with providers because of public pressure,[41] legislative initiatives,[42] and professional association action.[43]

Failure on the part of health care professionals to disclose to a patient any provider contractual financial incentives tied to providing less care evidences a lack of respect for patient autonomy. Patients have the right to receive all pertinent disclosure information related to their care. Is there any person who would not want to know that his or her health care provider is paid, in whole or in part, for saving money for the provider's employer by providing less care to the patient?

Summary

Informed patient consent to health care evaluation and treatment intervention is a legal and ethical prerequisite to care. Health care clinicians responsible for patient evaluation and treatment and intervention—especially rehabilitation professionals—bear primary responsibility for obtaining patient informed consent. Informed consent to rehabilitation intervention by nonphysician health care professionals is not the responsibility of referring physicians at one end of the continuum, nor of assistants or other supportive personnel carrying out the professionals' directives at the other end of the continuum.

Although the elements of legally sufficient patient informed consent vary from state to state (according to state or federal law, as applicable), the following

Compliance by providers with "gag clauses" in health professional employment contracts with managed care organizations may result in situations in which clinicians do not make full disclosure of treatment-related information to patients.

disclosure elements must normally be imparted to patients (or their surrogate decision makers) before health care commences:

- Diagnosis and pertinent evaluative findings
- Nature of the intervention(s) recommended or ordered
- Risk of potential harm or complications material to the patient's decision whether to accept or reject treatment
- Expected benefits (i.e., goals) of treatment
- Reasonable alternatives to the proposed treatment or intervention

In addition to the above disclosure elements, a health care professional must also solicit and satisfactorily answer any patient questions before the informed consent process is consummated. There is a variety of legally acceptable ways to document patient informed consent to treatment.

There are two principal exceptions to the requirement to obtain patient informed consent, the emergency doctrine and therapeutic privilege. In life-threatening emergency situations, it is generally presumed that patients grant implied consent to medical interventions designed to save their lives. (Exceptions to the exception may also apply, such as where a specific patient's prior contrary wishes are known.) Therapeutic privilege allows a physician to withhold diagnostic and/or prognostic information from a patient who is deemed to be psychologically incapable of dealing with the information. It is rarely allowed because the exception derogates from respect for patient autonomy and patient control over treatment-related decision making.

Human subject research informed consent is normally more formal and complex than patient informed consent, in part because of the substantial federal, state, and institutional oversight over human subject research activities, and in part, because of the (very recent) history of horrific abuse of human subjects in medical research. The details of the processes of human research subject informed consent are governed at the operative level by independent IRBs. There is a judicial trend to disallow nontherapeutic research posing greater than minimal health risks involving minors and incompetent subjects.

Managed care has given rise to informed consent practice issues, most involving actual or perceived provider conflicts of interest. The fundamental biomedical ethical principles of beneficence and respect for patient autonomy are in direct conflict with managed care contractual "gag clauses," which may prevent providers from making full disclosure of treatment-related information to patients and nondisclosure about provider financial incentives to provide less care to patients. The courts have yet to rule definitively on these issues but will likely declare these managed care initiatives unconscionable and unenforceable.

Cases and Questions

1. A physical therapist in private practice asks you for advice on the propriety of placing a rubber-stamped informed consent summary in each patient's treatment record to demonstrate that the patients have been provided with appropriate disclosure information and have, in fact, given informed consent to intervention. How do you advise the physical therapist?

2. As a facility risk manager, what steps can you take to ensure that rehabilitation professionals universally make appropriate disclosure of treatment-related information and obtain patient informed consent to intervention?

Suggested Answers for Cases and Questions

1. Informed consent is a communicative process and not a stamp or patient signature on a form.[44] A rubber-stamped summary of the information imparted to a patient might constitute some evidence of what was said to the patient but is normally unnecessary for routine interventions. Under managed care—where time is at a premium—the optimal method of documenting patient informed consent to intervention may be in a document such as a clinic policies and procedures manual or quality management manual, instead of placing individual documentation in patient treatment records for routine interventions. Health care providers will be expected by clinic managers, insurers, and the courts to universally comply with the institutional informed consent standards enunciated in such manuals.

2. Steps to ensure that providers carry out their legal and ethical duties related to disclosure of treatment-related information and the obtaining of patient informed consent include, among possible others:

   - Ensuring that newly employed providers read, and verify in writing, their understanding of the clinic policy regarding patient informed consent;
   - Monitoring selected patients for comprehension of disclosure information and consent to intervention[45]; and
   - Providing periodic in-service education, involving clinical professionals, ethicists, and legal counsel, on legal and ethical issues related to patient informed consent.

References

1. Beauchamp TL, Childress JF: *Principles of biomedical ethics,* ed 4, New York, 1994, Oxford Press.

2. In an early leading case on informed consent, *Schloendorf v. Society of New York Hospital,* 105 NE 2nd 92 (NY, 1914), Justice Benjamin Cardozo wrote, "Every human being of adult years and sound mind has a right to determine what shall be done with his [or her] own body, and a surgeon who performs an operation without [a] patient's consent commits an assault for which he [or she] is liable in money damages."

3. Katz J: *The silent world of doctor and patient,* New York, 1984, Free Press. "[D]isclosure and consent, except in the most rudimentary fashion, are obligations alien to medical thinking and practice."

4. Furrow BR, Johnson SH, Jost TS, Schwartz RL: *Health law: cases, materials and problems,* ed 2, St Paul, Minn, 1991, West Publishing, p 322.

5. See note 2.

6. *Natanson v. Kline,* 350 P.2d 1093 (Kansas, 1965).

7. *Canterbury v. Spence,* 464 F.2d 772 (Washington, DC, 1972), *cert.* [US Supreme Court appeal] *denied,* 409 US 1064, 1974.

8. American Physical Therapy Association: *Guide for professional conduct,* Section 1.4 (Informed Consent), Alexandria, Va, 1996, APTA.

9. American Occupational Therapy Association: *Occupational therapy code of ethics,* Principle 2B, Bethesda, Md, 1994, AOTA.

10. American Occupational Therapy Association: *Occupational therapy code of ethics,* Principle 2D, Bethesda, Md, 1994, AOTA.

11. *Schloendorf v. Society of New York Hospital.* See note 2.

12. "The fundamental distinction between assault and battery on one hand, and [professional] negligence such as would constitute malpractice, on the other, is that the former is intentional and the latter unintentional...." *Natanson v. Kline.* See note 2.

13. Furrow BR, Johnson SH, Jost TS, Schwartz RL: *Health law: cases, materials and problems,* ed 2, St Paul, Minn, 1991, West Publishing, p 327. See note 7, *Foflygen v. Zemel,* 615 A.2d 1345 (Pennsylvania, 1992).

14. Standards of Practice for Physical Therapy: *Informed consent,* provision of care, X. "The physical therapist obtains the patient's informed consent in accordance with jurisdictional law before initiating physical therapy." HOD Policy 06-91-21-25, Alexandria, Va, 1991, APTA.

15 *Spence v. Todaro,* No 94-3757 (ED Pa, 1994).

16. *Friter and Friter v. Iolab Corp.,* 607 A.2d 1111 (Pennsylvania Supreme Court, 1992).

17. *Flores v. Center for Spinal Evaluation and Rehabilitation,* 865 SW 2nd 261 (Tex App, 1993).

18. *In re* Quinlan, 355 A.2d 647 (NJ, 1976).

19. *Bouvia v. Superior Court,* 179 Calif App 3d 1127, 225 Calif Rptr 297 (Calif App, 1986).

20. *Cruzan v. Director,* Dept of Health, 110 S Ct,. 2841, 1990.

21. Patient Self-Determination Act, 42 United States Code Sections 1395, 1396.

22. 42 United States Code Section 1395cc(f)(1)(A)(i).

23. American Hospital Association: *Patient bill of rights and responsibilities,* Chicago, 1992, AHA.

24. Joint Commission on the Accreditation of Health Care Organizations: *Accreditation manual for hospitals,* Chicago, current edition, JCAHO.

25. *Canterbury v. Spence.* See note 7.

26. Curtin LL: Ethics in management: informed consent: cautious, calculated candor, *Nursing Management* 24(4):18, 1995.

27. How Is Your Doctor Treating You? *Consumer reports* 1995, p 81.

28. Tanner L: Study asks how much patients want to know, *Senior news* Oct 1995, p 15.

29. Furrow BR, Johnson SH, Jost TS, Schwartz RL: *Health law: cases, materials and problems,* ed 2, St Paul, Minn, 1991, West Publishing, p 336.

30. *Canterbury v. Spence.* See note 7.

31. American Medical Association, Council on Ethical and Judicial Affairs: Guidelines for the appropriate use of do-not-resuscitate orders, *JAMA* 265:1868, 1991.

32. Somerville MA: Therapeutic privilege: variation on the theme of informed consent, *Law, Medicine & Health Care* 12(1):4, 1984.

33. Searight HR: Assessing patient competence for medical decision making, *American Family Physician* 45:751, 1992.

34. Scott RW: *Legal aspects of documenting patient care,* Gaithersburg, Md, 1994, Aspen Publishers.

35. Principle 1, Nuremberg Code of 1947: *Trials of war criminals before the Nuremberg military tribunals under control council law no. 10,* vol 2, Washington, DC, 1949, US Government Printing Office, p 181.

36. World Medical Association Declaration of Helsinki: Principle 2, (Adopted by the 18th World Medical Assembly, Helsinki, Finland, 1964, and amended by the 29th World Medical Assembly, Tokyo, Japan, 1975) 35th World Medical Assembly, Venice, Italy, 1983 and 41st World Medical Assembly, Hong Kong, 1989.

37. Code of Federal Regulations: *Protection of human subjects,* Title 45, Part 46, Washington, DC, 1983, US Government Printing Office.

38. *TD v. New York State Office of Mental Health,* WL 695417 (N. App, 1996).

39. Barnes PG: Beyond Nuremberg, *ABA Journal* 83(3):24, 1997.

40. O'Brien C: *Memo: background and supporting documentation on gag clauses,* Chicago, 1995, American Medical Association, p 1.

41. Bursztajn HJ, Saunders LS, Brodsky A: Medical negligence and informed consent in the managed care era, *The Health Lawyer* 9(5):14, 1997.

42. McGinley L: Clinton to prohibit HMO gag clauses under Medicaid, *Wall Street Journal* Feb 20, 1997, p A22.

43. American Medical Association, Council on Ethical and Judicial Affairs: Ethical issues in managed care, *JAMA* 273:330, 1995.

44. Hudson T: Informed consent problems become more complicated, *Hospitals* Mar 20, 1991, pp 38-40.

45. Hutson MM, Blaha JD: Patients' recall of preoperative instruction for informed consent for an operation, *J Bone Joint Surg Am* 73A:160, 1991.

Suggested Readings

American Hospital Association: *Patient bill of rights and responsibilities,* Chicago, 1992, AHA.

American Medical Association, Council on Ethical and Judicial Affairs: Ethical issues in managed care, *JAMA* 273:330, 1995.

American Occupational Therapy Association: *Occupational therapy code of ethics,* Bethesda, Md, 1994, AOTA.

American Physical Therapy Association: *Guide for professional conduct,* Section 1.4 (Informed Consent), Alexandria, Va, 1996, APTA.

Barnes PG: Beyond Nuremberg, *ABA Journal* 83(3):24, 1997.

Beauchamp TL, Childress JF: *Principles of biomedical ethics,* ed 4, New York, 1994, Oxford Press.

Bursztajn HJ, Saunders LS, Brodsky A: Medical negligence and informed consent in the managed care era, *The Health Lawyer* 9(5):14, 1997.

Canterbury v. Spence, 464 F.2d 772 (Washington, DC, 1972), *cert.* [US Supreme Court appeal] *denied,* 409 US 1064, 1974.

Code of Federal Regulations: *Protection of human subjects,* Title 45, Part 46, Washington, DC, 1983, US Government Printing Office.

Curtin LL: Ethics in management: informed consent: cautious, calculated candor, *Nursing Management* 24(4):18, 1995.

Furrow BR, Johnson SH, Jost TS, Schwartz RL: *Health law: cases, materials and problems,* ed 2, St Paul, Minn, 1991, West Publishing, p 336.

How Is Your Doctor Treating You? *Consumer reports* Feb 1995, p 81.

Hutson MM, Blaha JD: Patients' recall of preoperative instruction for informed consent for an operation, *J Bone Joint Surg Am* 73A:160, 1991.

Hudson T: Informed consent problems become more complicated, *Hospitals* Mar 20, 1991, pp 38-40.

Joint Commission on the Accreditation of Health Care Organizations: *Accreditation manual for hospitals,* Chicago, 1997, JCAHO.

Journal of the American Physical Therapy Association: Guidelines for physical therapy documentation, *J Am Phys Ther Assoc* 75:762, 1995.

Katz J: *The silent world of doctor and patient,* New York, 1984, Free Press.

McGinley L: Clinton to prohibit HMO gag clauses under medicaid, *Wall Street Journal* A22, 1997.

O'Brien C: *Memo: background and supporting documentation on gag clauses,* Chicago, 1995, American Medical Association, p 1.

Patient Self-Determination Act, 42 United States Code Sections 1395, 1396.

Portney LG, Watkins MP: *Foundations of clinical research: applications to practice,* Norwalk, Conn, 1993, Appleton & Lange, p 27.

Rozovsky FA: *Consent to treatment,* ed 2, Boston, 1990, Little, Brown.

Scott RW: *Legal aspects of documenting patient care,* Gaithersburg, Md, 1994, Aspen Publishers.

Searight HR: Assessing patient competence for medical decision making, *American Family Physician* 45:751, 1992.

Somerville MA: Therapeutic privilege: variation on the theme of informed consent, *Law, Medicine & Health Care* 12(1):4, 1984.

Tanner L: Study asks how much patients want to know, *Senior news* Oct 1995, p 15.

Timm K: Informed consent in clinical research, *Orthopaedic Practice* 7(3):14, 1995.

Winslow R: Videos, questionnaires aim to expand role of patients in treatment decisions, *Wall Street Journal* Feb 25,1992, p B1.

Professional Practice Issues

This chapter addresses the ethical aspects of several important health professional practice issues, initially including the privileges and responsibilities of professional licensure and certification, the nature of practice acts and governing administrative regulations, customary practice, practice settings and arrangements, and clinical specialization. Next, this chapter explores ethical questions involving relations among health professionals and professions and cross-training and multiskilling initiatives. Ethical issues related to financial responsibilities of providers and patients are addressed, as is the nature of *pro bono publico* health care service, using the legal profession as a suggested model for emulation. This chapter concludes with discussion of confidentiality of patient, proprietary and peer-review information; the ethical duties of providers of fidelity and truthfulness; and ethical concerns regarding accepting and giving gifts related to official health professional duties.

●

Licensure and Certification

Licensure and/or certification, like academic degrees and other relevant credentials, are indicators of special professional status under law. The processes of licensure and certification create exclusive or primary domains of practice. The privileges of licensure and certification give licensees and certificants the exclusive, or at least the primary, right to practice their professions.

There is a growing number of licensed professions, and the process of licensure is under legislative attack. Certain health professionals—including physicians and surgeons, dentists, registered and licensed practical nurses, physical and occupational therapists and assistants, and chiropractors, among others—are subject to mandatory licensure requirements for professional practice.

The licensure of professionals is within the exclusive domain of the states and does not reside with the federal government. The processes of establishing standards for and granting and administering licenses, and disciplining licensed professions are an exercise of states' Tenth Amendment federal constitutional "police power" (i.e., the power to maintain order and discipline and to promote public health and safety and the general welfare, within the borders of the state.[1]

If licensure is mandatory to practice a profession within a state, the state requiring licensure can forbid unlicensed persons—even those qualified to practice through education and licensure in other states—to practice within the state until they fulfill the reasonable licensure requirements of that particular state. For health professionals licensed in another state, state governmental licensure agencies typically grant temporary licensure for those professionals to practice within a state for a limited period of time pending completion of instate licensure requirements. It is common among the health professions for states to grant licensure to professionals licensed in other states via reciprocity. For other professions, however—particularly the legal profession—licensure by reciprocity may not be the norm, particularly in heavily populated "sunbelt" states.

Loco tenems (Latin for "holding the place") is a form of temporary licensure granted by a state to an individual health care professional licensed in another state for a fixed period of time (e.g., "for a period not to exceed 6 months.") Traveling health care professionals commonly practice their itinerant professions in multiple states through *loco tenems* temporary licensure.

It is unethical and illegal for a health professional licensed in one state to practice his or her profession in a state in which he or she is unlicensed and in which professional licensure is mandatory. It is similarly unlawful and unethical for a health professional licensed to practice one profession to engage in the unlicensed practice of another health profession. The unlicensed practice of a licensed health profession is usually a violation of the administrative, civil, and criminal laws of a state, as well as a breach of professional ethics.

The privileges of licensure and certification give licensees and certificants the exclusive, or at least the primary, right to practice their professions.

72

The earliest reported legal cases involving physical therapy in the United States involved criminal charges brought by district attorneys for the unlicensed practice of medicine by physical therapists and extenders. For example, in *People v. Mari*,[2] a New York case from 1933, a physical therapist was convicted of the unlicensed practice of medicine incident to the treatment of a rheumatism patient. Similarly, in *People v. Dennis*,[3] another New York case from 1946, a masseur employed by a physical therapist was convicted of the unlicensed practice of medicine.

Mandatory licensure laws governing health care professional practice are subject to periodic "zero-base" review[4] pursuant to *sunset review*[5] of their provisions by state legislatures. Health professionals are presumed by law to have *constructive knowledge* of the provisions of the licensure laws and implementing administrative regulations governing their official activities.

Practice Acts and Governmental Regulations

State statutory licensure laws and implementing regulatory practice acts define the parameters of licensed health professional practice. These parameters include, among other considerations:

- Requirements for licensure of United States–educated professionals
- Requirements for licensure of foreign-trained professionals
- Requirements for continuing professional education
- Requirements for practice within the state pursuant to temporary licensure
- Requirements for periodic relicensure
- Requirements for mandatory reporting of perceived unethical conduct scope of permissible practice
- Restrictions, if any, on independent or autonomous practice ("practice without referral")
- Provisions addressing *sunset review*, if any
- Provisions establishing licensure boards to administer professional licensure
- Provisions defining grounds and procedures for disciplinary action

In addition to being violations of professional ethical standards, violations of mandatory licensure laws designed to protect public health and safety are punishable as criminal offenses and form the basis for administrative claims and civil health care malpractice lawsuits. In civil malpractice litigation incident to unlicensed health professional practice, a defendant is normally held to the legal standard of care of a licensed professional in the discipline in which unlicensed practice has occurred.

The Tenth Amendment grants states the power to maintain order and discipline and to promote public health and safety and the general welfare, within the borders of the state.

Customary Practice

Whereas licensure laws and their implementing practice acts, other governmental regulations, and certification standards establish the general framework for discipline-specific health professional practice, the residuum of the *standard of care* derives from customary practice methods and patterns. No licensure law, practice act, or system of certification standards can be reasonably expected to define in detail the complex minutiae of health professional practice.

It is self-evident that customary health professional practice is normally relied upon to establish a health discipline's legal standard of care in legal proceedings. This fact is reflected in the extensive use of expert witnesses in health care malpractice proceedings to testify for patients, providers, and the state about whether, in retrospect, care rendered by a health care professional fell within or below minimally acceptable practice standards. If documented practice standards were always sufficient to establish the legal health professional standard of care and the violation thereof, then expert witness testimony would be unnecessary in health care malpractice legal cases, as is usually the case in *ordinary negligence* cases, such as those involving slips and falls by clients on defendants' premises.

Many or most health care professionals will be called upon, during their careers, to render expert testimony in legal proceedings. It is imperative, therefore, to understand the essence of a health care expert witness.

The overwhelming majority of decisions in health care malpractice legal cases is strongly influenced by expert witness testimony. Health professional expert witnesses, testifying for patients or professional colleagues, may be asked to testify concerning the following considerations, among others: patient evaluation, treatment, and product design; use of therapeutic modalities and equipment; discipline-specific informed consent processes; and referral and consultation statutory and customary practice. A health professional expert specifically opines about whether a health professional–defendant's care of a patient met or violated minimally acceptable practice standards for the health care discipline represented by the defendant.

To be *legally competent* to testify as an expert, a witness must meet two basic requirements:

- The expert must be knowledgeable concerning the health professional product or service at issue in the case.
- The expert must be familiar—directly or indirectly—with the legal standard of care (i.e., relevant laws and customs) for the defendant's health care discipline at the time that the incident creating the legal controversy arose.

An expert's credentials must be established by the attorney representing the party using the testimony of the expert witness. Any expert witness is subject to challenge through impeachment by opposing legal counsel. In many civil and criminal cases, judges and lay juries are asked to weigh the relative credibility of competing expert witnesses for plaintiffs and defendants and reach decisions based on their best judgments.

Who can testify for or against defendant–health care professionals in legal cases? In some jurisdictions, prospective experts are required to hold the same academic credentials as the defendant-provider, under the "same school," of same-discipline legal doctrine. In other jurisdictions, experts merely must be qualified under the same criteria of knowledge of the product or service in issue and familiarity with the applicable legal standard of care at the time of occurrence of the incident.

There are certain ethical duties incumbent upon an expert witness. Experts must carefully evaluate the facts of the cases and render accurate and objective professional opinions. An expert must not display an attitudinal bias toward one side in a case. If this occurs, the expert will lose credibility with all process participants—parties, judge, and jury—involved in the legal proceeding, as well as with professional colleagues.

Health care professionals should not decline an invitation to serve as expert witnesses in legal proceedings. If subject-matter health professional experts do not come forward to testify on behalf of patients, peers, and others, the goal of a just result might not be achieved. Providers should consider expert witness testimony like any other civic duty, including voting, jury duty, and registering for military service, as required by law.

Practice Settings and Arrangements

Rehabilitation and other health care professionals are employed in the widest range of variegated practice settings. Largely, rehabilitation professional practice has transitioned over time from what was formerly a hospital-based inpatient practice setting to practice that takes place in hospital, outpatient clinical, school, work place, home, long-term care, and other settings.

In all practice settings, health care professionals have the ethical duty to recognize patients' right of freedom of choice in selection of health care providers.[6,7] This right seemingly has become eroded under the managed care paradigm, where patients choose their health care professionals from restricted lists of eligible providers. However, health care professionals must still be respectful of this fundamental patient right, within the parameters of the contractual care plan of a particular patient.

It is critical that health care professionals interacting with patients and clients in these settings be cognizant of their special needs, particularly the legitimate privacy interests of patients and clients. It is a relative challenge in hospital and outpatient clinical settings to provide a modicum of privacy for patients; however, it must

Health care professionals have the ethical duty to recognize patients' right of freedom of choice in selecting health care providers, which seemingly has become eroded under the managed care paradigm, where patients choose their health care professionals from restricted lists of eligible providers.

75

be done to the extent feasible. The same consideration applies to care rendered in other settings—such as in patients' homes—where patient privacy is relatively easier to maintain.

A mundane, but important, patient privacy consideration is the need for appropriate draping during evaluation and treatment.[8] By expending special effort to respect patient modesty by minimizing the exposure of body parts and surface areas during evaluation and treatment, health care providers demonstrate respect for patient autonomy, enhance patient cooperation with evaluative and treatment procedures, and perhaps reduce patients' allegations of health care malpractice and unethical conduct.

Multidisciplinary and interdisciplinary health professional group practices have become commonplace in recent years and are particularly prominent under managed care, where cost containment is a coprimary objective, along with optimal quality patient care services and products. Rehabilitation health professional codes of ethics reflect that these group practice arrangements are generally ethically acceptable. For example, Section 5.2C of the *Guide for Professional Conduct*[6] of the American Physical Therapy Association states that:

> Physical therapists may enter into agreements with organizations to provide physical therapy services if such agreements do not violate the ethical principles of the Association.

Similarly, Section 4.2 of the *Canons of Ethical Conduct*[7] of the American Board for Certification in Orthotics and Prosthetics, concerning ancillary commercial services, states that:

> [T]he orthotist or prosthetist is not prohibited from providing related commercial services, such as furnishing...durable medical supplies, as long as the patient and the public in general are made aware of the differences between the orthotist's and prosthetist's professional and commercial services.

Although this subject might not be specifically addressed in other rehabilitation health professional ethics codes, the provisions of ancillary services, such as marketing supplies to patients in clinical practice, is generally not prohibited, unless their sale is the result of fraud, deception, or overreaching.

Clinical Specialization

Clinical specialization evidences advanced competency practice, in the eyes of professional peers, patients, and the public-at-large. The objectives of the American Physical Therapy Association's American Board of Physical Therapy Specialties program objectives typify those of related disciplines and seek:

...to promote the highest possible level of care for individuals seeking...services in each specialty area; to assist consumers, the health community, and others in identifying certified clinical specialists in each specialty area; and to promote the development of the science and the art of each specialty area of practice.[9]

The American Board of Physical Therapy Specialties certifies clinical specialists in the following practice areas:

- Cardiopulmonary
- Clinical electrophysiologic
- Geriatric
- Neurologic
- Orthopedic
- Pediatric
- Sports

Occupational therapist–advanced competency practitioners may be certified by the American Occupational Therapy Association in two areas, pediatrics and neurologic rehabilitation.[10] Rehabilitation nurses may be certified by the Association of Rehabilitation Nurses as Certified Rehabilitation Registered Nurses.[11] Orthotists and prosthetists are not currently certified in specialty practice areas.

Other professional associations and entities, such as the American Hand Society and the McKenzie Institute, among others, offer clinical specialty certification to rehabilitation professionals. It is unethical to misrepresent one's credentials to patients, professional colleagues, employers, and others. Those rehabilitation professionals who engage in specialized practice, but are not certified as clinical specialists, should apprise patients and others of the distinction to prevent any misunderstanding of a provider's credentials. (In legal practice, such a potential misunderstanding on the part of clients is obviated in states such as Texas, where non–certified-specialist attorneys are required to annotate on their official correspondence and calling cards that they are "not certified by the Texas Board of Legal Certification."[12])

Relations Among Health Care Professions and Professionals

Professional relations within and among health care disciplines generally have been consistently positive over time. There are, however, professional ethical issues involving intradisciplinary and interdisciplinary health professional relations that bear mentioning.

In recent times, millions of dollars in legal fees have been spent prosecuting or defending intradisciplinary and interdisciplinary encroachment or "turf" or jurisdictional battles between or among complementary health professional disciplines or organizations. Issues addressed in these legal battles range from use of terminology to domains of practice to credentialing to antitrust.

In perhaps the most prominent of these legal cases, *Wilk v. American Medical Association,*[13] a federal appellate court ruled that the medical community had carried out an illegal boycott of the chiropractic profession in violation of Section One of the Sherman Antitrust Act of 1890.[14]

Health professionals, individually and collectively, and health professional organizations should consider resolving such disputes in a more amicable manner than through civil litigation. These groups should consider utilizing alternative dispute resolution methods, including third-party mediation and arbitration. In *mediation,* a neutral third-party intermediary facilitates a mutually agreeable solution to a dispute by the parties themselves. In *arbitration,* a neutral third party conducts the administrative equivalent of a private civil legal proceeding and renders a decision, to which the parties to the dispute contractually agree to be bound. Under either method of alternative dispute resolution, a public record of proceedings is avoided, the cost of dispute resolution in terms of time and money is reduced, and professional goodwill may be enhanced.

Rehabilitation professional codes of ethics address intradisciplinary and interdisciplinary relations directly and indirectly. Perhaps the most direct reference to this topic is found in Section 1.1C of the *Guide for Professional Conduct* of the American Physical Therapy Association, which reads:

> Physical therapists shall not engage in conduct that constitutes harassment or abuse of, or discrimination against, colleagues, associates, or others.

Multiskilling and Cross-Training Initiatives

The era of managed care, with its dual emphases on cost containment and efficiency in health care delivery, has created strong interest in creating multiskilled rehabilitation professionals and extender personnel. In its *Third Report,*[15] the Pew Health Professions Commission specifically recommended that allied health professional education programs focus on interdisciplinary core curricula and multiskilling.

Cross training may be defined as the preparation of a health care provider to perform functions associated with another discipline. A *multiskilled* health care provider is one who has demonstrated competence in the skill sets of more than one health professional discipline.

The areas of multiskilling and cross training of health care professionals involve intensely interwoven law and ethical considerations. State practice acts of particular health professional disciplines may make expressly unlawful encroachment by unlicensed providers upon the applicable delineated domain of practice. Practice

State practice acts may make expressly unlawful encroachment by unlicensed providers upon the applicable delineated domain of practice. Practice acts and health professional codes of ethics spell out requirements for supervision of assistant professionals and unlicensed extender personnel.

78

acts and health professional codes[16-19] of ethics spell out requirements for supervision of assistant professionals and unlicensed extender personnel.

The Association of Rehabilitation Nurses has promulgated a position paper entitled, *The Role of Unlicensed Assistive Personnel in the Rehabilitation Setting*,[20] which spells out basic and advanced, or "secondary," scope of care activities deemed appropriate for unlicensed assistive nursing personnel. Policy makers in other rehabilitation disciplines should review this paper for possible adaptation to their professions in a manner consistent with legal and ethical mandates and guidance.

Financial Responsibility: Ethical Duties of Patients and Providers

Patient Duty to Pay Fair Value for Professional Services

Patients are not bound by a formal code of ethical conduct in their relations with health care professionals, as are the latter. However, certain legal duties are incumbent upon patients receiving treatment in health care delivery settings. The principle duty of patients (absent legal excusal or release by the provider) is to pay market or fair value for professional services rendered. This legal obligation is the primary duty of patients cited by authorities as creating legal *consideration* under the implied health care professional–patient contractual relationship. (The principle legal duty incumbent upon the provider is, of course, to exercise his or her best clinical judgment to affect an optimal therapeutic result for the patient.)

Health Care Professionals' Duties

Pricing of Services. Health care organizations—whether operated for-profit or not-for-profit—are businesses and must normally generate sufficient operating revenue (absent receipt of subsidies, donations, or investment or other nonoperating revenue) to cover the direct and indirect costs of patient care. Direct costs include salaries for professional and support staff and supplies and equipment used in patient care activities. Indirect costs include, among others, employee benefits, administrative and maintenance expenses, depreciation on equipment, and housekeeping and laundry expenses.[21]

The processes associated with pricing of health care services and products give rise to potential ethical problems, issues, and dilemmas for health care providers and administrators. Managed care and prospective payment systems (PPS) have given rise to discounted and fixed reimbursement for inpatient and outpatient health services.

Representative rehabilitation health care professional codes of ethics address the pricing of professional services as follows:

Sections 3.5 and 3.6 of the *Canons of Ethical Conduct* of the American

Patients are not bound by a formal code of ethical conduct in their relations with health care professionals. The principle legal duty incumbent upon the provider is to exercise his or her best clinical judgment to affect an optimal therapeutic result for the patient.

Board for Certification in Orthotics and Prosthetics address professional fees in a most comprehensive manner. Section 3.5 (Fees and Compensation) reads:

> Fees for orthotic and prosthetic services should be reasonable for the services performed, taking into consideration the setting in which the services are provided, the practice costs in the geographic area, the judgment of other related and similar organizations, and other relevant factors. The orthotist and prosthetist shall never place his or her own financial interest above the welfare of the patient. It is unethical for the orthotist or prosthetist to engage in false, misleading or deceptive actions in relation to the ultimate cost of services undertaken or furnished. Over utilization caused by continuing orthotics or prosthetics services beyond the point of possible benefit or by providing services more frequently than necessary is unethical.

Submission of false or misleading information in requesting reimbursement from third-party payers, including Medicare and private insurers, is unethical.

Section 3.6 (Practice Arrangements) imposes a lofty ethical standard for beneficence upon orthotists and prosthetists. It reads in pertinent part:

> The orthotist and prosthetist *shall* [emphasis added] refer all patients to the most cost beneficial service provider, taking into consideration the nature and extent of the problem, treatment resources and availability of health care benefit coverage, and the likelihood of receiving appropriate and beneficial care.

Sections 5.1 and 5.2 of the *Guide for Professional Conduct* of the American Physical Therapy Association address fees and fee arrangements. Section 5.1 (Fiscally Sound Remuneration) reads:

> A. Physical therapists shall never place their own financial interests above the welfare of individuals under their care.
> B. Fees for physical therapy services should be reasonable for the service performed, considering the setting in which it is provided, practice costs in the geographic area, judgment of other organizations and other relevant factors.
> C. Physical therapists should attempt to ensure that providers, agencies, or other employers adopt physical therapy fee schedules that are reasonable and that encourage access to necessary services.

Section 5.2B (Business Practices/Fee Arrangements) reads:

> Unless laws impose restrictions to the contrary, physical therapists who provide physical therapy services in a business entity may pool fees and monies received. Physical therapists may divide or apportion these fees and monies in accordance with the business arrangement.

Principle 1D of the *Occupational Therapy Code of Ethics* reads:

Occupational therapy personnel shall strive to ensure that fees are fair, reasonable, and commensurate with the service performed and are set with due regard for the service recipient's ability to pay.

The common thread of "reasonableness" among the rehabilitation professional ethics codes in setting fees is augmented by the implied principle that fees for professional rehabilitation services must also be "realistic"; that is, fees for professional services must be set high enough to generate sufficient net income for the rehabilitation professional to enjoy a fair living standard commensurate with his or her labor efforts and level of education and experience.

Under managed care, many rehabilitation professionals deliver care under contractual capitation arrangements. Under *capitation,* providers agree to provide all necessary professional services to program subscribers (patients) for a fixed fee, often expressed as "per member per month" (PMPM).[22] Before entering into capitation arrangements, rehabilitation professionals should consult their legal counsel and financial advisor; conduct a relevant market analysis; and ensure that projected revenues under the contract will exceed projected expenses, so that established fees are both reasonable and realistic.

Maintaining Professional and General Liability Insurance. Health care professional–business owners may be claimed against, or sued, by patients, business licensees on the premises, employees, contractors, visitors, and others for injuries that are the result of a breach of a legal duty owed by the health care professional–business owner to them, such as failure to maintain safe premises. Such *premises liability,* a form of *ordinary negligence,* is the kind that can occur on any business premises and therefore is not health care malpractice, for which practice-related sanctions may ensue.

Health care professionals also may be claimed against, or sued, by patients or their legal representatives for treatment-related health care malpractice. A settlement or adverse judgment against a health care professional for malpractice carries with it practice-related sanctions, including possible inclusion of the provider's name in the National Practitioner Data Bank, a health care malpractice database maintained by the federal government, which is open to licensure entities and employers.

Health care employers and business owners are required to provide (and pay for) unemployment compensation and (in most cases) workers' compensation insurance. Normally required by law, health care employers and business owners are also expected to carry sufficient professional and general liability insurance to cover foreseeable potential losses.

Fees for professional services must be set high enough to generate sufficient net income for the rehabilitation professional to enjoy a fair living standard commensurate with his or her labor efforts and level of education and experience.

81

For businesses that are incorporated, business owners normally enjoy the right to liability limited to their investments in the enterprise. However, courts have occasionally "pierced the corporate veil" to impose unlimited personal liability upon corporate officers and owners when judges find that such corporations have unethically undercapitalized or underinsured their businesses against foreseeable potential losses.

Pro Bono Publico Service to Socioeconomically Disadvantaged Patients

When professional service is provided *pro bono publico* (Latin for "for the public good"), it is provided either at a reduced fee or for no fee, depending on the ability of the service recipient to pay. For rehabilitation professionals who participate in *pro bono* activities, the benefits are both tangible and intangible.

The public image of an individual provider, his or her business organization, and his or her profession are all enhanced through a strong commitment to public service. Both personal and collective satisfaction result when professionals respond to a compelling need for the profession's services. In addition, improvement in a business entity's goodwill of an organization enhances revenue and/or profit; a network is created among colleagues performing similar services; and professional associations and public entities provide technical and administrative support that ensures overall success of *pro bono* efforts.[23]

Regardless of these considerations, the ethical and legal responsibility of rehabilitation professionals to patients lacking the ability to pay for services is an area of concern and confusion. Section 8.1 of the *Guide for Professional Conduct* of the American Physical Therapy Association and Principle 1D of the *Occupational Therapy Code of Ethics* provide guidance for all health care professionals concerning *pro bono* ethical obligations:

Section 8.1 (Pro Bono Service) of the *Guide for Professional Conduct* of the American Physical Therapy Association reads:

> Physical therapists should render pro bono publico (reduced or no fee) services to patients lacking the ability to pay for services, as each physical therapist's practice permits.

Principle 1D of the Occupational Therapy Code of Ethics reads in pertinent part:

> Occupational therapy personnel shall strive to ensure that fees are...set with due regard for the service recipient's ability to pay.

Both personal and collective satisfaction result when professionals respond to a compelling need for the profession's services.

In Search of a Model for *Pro Bono* Service

Of all the professions, the legal profession may have the most extensive documented history of pro bono service and expectations. In fact, *pro bono* professional service in the United States has traditionally focused on the legal profession. Many of the *pro bono* concepts utilized by the legal profession may be directly transferable to the health professions.

The legal profession has a century-old commitment to provide legal services to people who cannot afford them. In the twentieth century, this altruistic goal was formalized into a canon of ethical conduct by the American Bar Association in its *Canons of Professional Ethics* (1908),[24] the *Model Code of Professional Responsibility* (1969),[25] and the *Model Rules of Professional Conduct* (1983).[26] Although the original *Canons of Professional Ethics* made pro bono service mandatory for attorneys, the *Model Code and Model Rules*—adopted by the state bars of all 50 states—label attorneys' *pro bono* service obligation as an "ethical," rather than a "legal," obligation.

In its Rule 6.1 of the *Model Rules of Professional Conduct*, the American Bar Association established the following professional ethical standard for attorneys regarding *pro bono* service:

> A lawyer *should* [emphasis added] render public interest legal service. A lawyer may discharge this responsibility by providing professional services at no fee or at a reduced fee to persons of limited means or to public service or charitable groups or organizations, by services in activities for improving the law, the legal system or the legal profession, and by financial support for organizations that provide legal services to persons of limited means.

The nonbinding "Comment" to Rule 6.1 of the *Model Rules of Professional Conduct* expounds on this ethical principle by stating:

> Every lawyer, regardless of professional prominence or professional work load, should find time to participate in or otherwise support the provision of legal services to the disadvantaged. The provision of free legal services to those unable to pay reasonable fees continues to be an obligation of each lawyer, as well as the profession generally.

Rocky Road of Commitment

At the National Conference on Access to Justice in the 1990s, held in June 1989 in New Orleans, Lardent[27] sketched out the inconsistent history of attorney commitment to *pro bono* activity, emphasizing that the current *pro bono* involvement was meeting only about 20 percent of the legal services needs of the socioeconomically disadvantaged population. Lardent attributed much of the blame to professional associations, which she believed failed to: (1) take the lead in institutionalizing *pro bono* service as a practice expectation; (2) integrate *pro bono* programs into professional services and establish normative standards and assessment criteria; and (3) offer technical assistance to volunteers. Lardent pointed out, however, that several state bar associations were contemplating making mandatory a *de minimis* amount of *pro bono* service as a condition for licensure.

Several state court systems and the federal government have experimented with mandatory *pro bono* legal services. One justification for such a requirement is the argument that, because attorneys enjoy a virtual monopoly on the practice of law, they owe a public duty to represent, at a reduced fee or free of charge, clients who are indigent. Another more altruistic justification is based on the belief that representation of all clients before courts of law is an ethical, professional, and social responsibility of licensed attorneys.[28] (Cannot the same considerations be applied to rehabilitation health care professionals?)

In 1992 the Florida State Bar Association enacted a regulation that came very close to mandating universal *pro bono* service for Florida-licensed attorneys. The regulation established the expectation that Florida-licensed attorneys would perform a minimum of 20 hours of voluntary *pro bono* legal services annually or make a cash contribution of $350 to help defray the cost of providing legal services to the poor. The Florida regulation also required state-licensed attorneys to report their *pro bono* service to the state on an annual basis. This system of service and reporting was validated by the Florida Supreme Court as legal.[29] Other states, including Texas, have adopted similar plans for reporting *pro bono* services and for contributing monetarily to *pro bono* legal services for the poor.

Health care professional associations and state and federal regulatory agencies have offered relatively few *pro bono* guidelines.

Health Professions and *Pro Bono* Service

With 37 million Americans uninsured or underinsured for health care and a quarter of the population over 65 years of age living below the poverty line,[30] there is obviously a tremendous need for *pro bono* health care in the United States. Some of this need is currently being met by individuals and groups; however, health care professional associations and state and federal regulatory agencies have offered relatively few *pro bono* guidelines.

Legislators and health policy makers have created, or have attempted to create, various incentives to encourage health care professionals to engage in *pro bono* activities. Several states provide a type of "good Samaritan" immunity from health care malpractice liability for health care professionals performing *pro bono* services. This statutory immunity protects health care providers from liability so long as the providers' conduct does not constitute gross negligence, recklessness, or willful misconduct. The American Tort Reform has been lobbying for nationwide uniform protection for health care professionals in all practice settings to encourage greater participation in *pro bono* activities on the part of providers.[31]

Federal legislators have also introduced various bills that would statutorily relieve the nation's 200,000 federally funded care clinics treating indigent patients from paying health care malpractice insurance premiums. Under these proposals (and similar ones introduced in state legislatures), clinicians in such facilities would be treated as governmental employees (agents), thus immunizing them from personal malpractice liability exposure. (Under the Federal Tort Claims Act of 1949 and the Federal Employees Liability Reform and Tort Compensation Act of 1988, the federal government assumes vicarious liability and financial responsibility for health care malpractice settlements and court judgments involving federal employees.[32])

Fear of Health Care Malpractice Liability as a Barrier to Greater *Pro Bono* Service

Fear of liability exposure prevents many health care professionals engaged in clinical service delivery from providing *pro bono* services. Part of the fear stems from the belief that, because patients with low incomes may be more prone to adverse care outcomes because of relatively poor baseline health, they will more likely file claims against, or sue, their health care providers. Federal studies have reached different conclusions regarding the correlation between socioeconomic status and patient propensity to file a claim against, or sue, a health care provider. One 1991 Maryland study concluded that obstetric Medicaid patients showed no greater likelihood than women in general to file medical malpractice claims against their obstetricians.[33]

One way to dampen a provider's fear of malpractice liability exposure incident to *pro bono* service activities would be the creation of a legislative exception by Congress to the mandatory reporting requirements of the National Practitioner Data Bank. Designed in part to serve as a resource for verifying the accuracy of information provided by licensed health care professional job applicants to employers, the National Practitioner Data Bank also requires "health care institutions, boards of medical examiners, professional societies of medical doctors, dentists, and other health care practitioners, and malpractice payment entities to report malpractice payments."[34]

Besides legislative initiatives, health care professionals can take affirmative clinical risk management steps to minimize potential malpractice liability exposure. Simple initiatives, including effective communication with patients and their significant others; empathy; good rapport; and accurate, timely documentation of patient evaluation and care go a long way in protecting providers from liability.[35]

Simple initiatives, including effective communication with patients and their significant others; empathy; good rapport; and accurate, timely documentation of patient evaluation and care, go a long way in protecting providers from liability.

Pro Bono Publico Service: A Social Responsibility

All health professionals and professional associations, clinical entities, and academic health centers should carefully examine the model for *pro bono* service established by the legal profession and consider implementing minimally intrusive *pro bono* service expectations of members, employees, faculty, and staff, as applicable. State agencies, which license primary health care providers—including physicians, physical and occupational therapists, nurse practitioners, physician assistants, and others—should consider codifying *pro bono* expectations into law in the form of rules and regulations in state practice acts.

In addition to establishing *pro bono* policies, professional associations, clinical sites and universities, and state and federal agencies must assume responsibility for integrating *pro bono* efforts across all health care disciplines, providing continuing education, networking, and administrative and other support for volunteers who give their time to help socioeconomically disadvantaged clients. Professional corporations, practice groups, and individual providers also may consider incorporating *pro bono* policies into their practices and publicizing their *pro bono* efforts to encourage and provide guidance to others.[36-38]

Pro bono service should be an expectation—never a requirement—of all professionals to whom the states have granted the exclusive right to practice professions for profit. The tangible and intangible benefits to patients served, volunteer providers, practice groups, professional associations and professions, and society at large are limitless.

Confidentiality

The duty of confidentiality concerning patient health-related information is a mixed ethical and legal duty—one that is imposed both by health professional codes of ethics and by law, in professional practice acts and in other governing statutes and regulations. The duty incumbent upon a health care professional to safeguard confidential information extends, too, to proprietary business information belonging to employers, partnerships, and other business entities. As has been stated previously (see Chapter 3), where duties owed to patients and employers come into conflict, the provider's paramount duty is to patients under his or her care.

Patient Information

The ethical duty to safeguard confidential patient information is at least as old as the Hippocratic Oath, wherein it is stated:

> That whatsoever you shall see or hear of the lives of men (or women) which is not fitting to be spoken, you will keep inviolably secret.

The ethical duty to safeguard confidential patient information is at least as old as the Hippocratic Oath.

Each of the representative ethical codes for the rehabilitation professions also addresses the fundamental ethical principle of patient confidentiality. For example, Section 3.1 (Confidential Information) of the *Canons of Ethical Conduct* of the American Board for Certification in Orthotics and Prosthetics states that:

> All information relating to a patient's background, condition, treatment, management plan or any other information relating to the orthotist or prosthetist–patient relationship is and shall always remain confidential and may not be communicated to any third party not involved in the patient's care without the prior written consent of the patient or the patient's legal guardian.
>
> The confidentiality requirements...shall be strictly adhered to by all certificants unless the information is required by court order or when it is necessary to disclose such information to protect the welfare of the patient and/or the community. In such event, all disclosures shall be in accordance with applicable legal requirements.

Section 1.2 (Confidential Information) of the Guide for Professional Conduct of the American Physical Therapy Association reads:

> A. Information relating to the physical therapist-patient relationship is confidential and may not be communicated to a third party not involved in that patient's care without the prior written consent of the patient, subject to applicable law.
> D. Information may be disclosed to appropriate authorities when it is necessary to protect the welfare of an individual or the community. Such disclosure shall be in accordance with applicable law.

Sections 2.2 and 2.3 of the *Guide for Conduct of the Affiliate Member* of the American Physical Therapy Association state that:

> 2.2. Physical therapist assistants shall refer all requests for release of confidential information to the supervising physical therapist.
> 2.3 Physical therapist assistants must treat as confidential all information relating to the personal conditions and affairs of the persons whom they serve.

Principle 2E of the *Occupational Therapy Code of Ethics* reads:

> Occupational therapy personnel shall protect the confidential nature of information gained from educational, practice, research, and investigational activities.

As these ethical provisions imply, the supervising licensed or certified health professional is primarily responsible for his or her conduct related to maintaining patient confidences and for ensuring that all persons under his or her direction safeguard confidential patient information. These health care professionals include students and volunteers, who may not have had prior acclimatization to the sensitivity of maintaining patient information as confidential. Consider the following example (based on an actual incident):

> Two health-career high school student volunteers are working in the Sexually Transmitted Disease Section of ABC Hospital's Clinical Laboratory Services Department. A physical therapy staff member overhears them in the medical library, discussing the HIV status of an identified patient. What should the physical therapist do?
>
> The physical therapist should immediately intervene and direct the two volunteers to cease publicizing confidential information concerning the patient. The therapist should apprise them of the nature of confidentiality; take their names and report the incident to the supervisor of the Sexually Transmitted Disease Section and to the hospital's risk manager by filing an incident report. Breach of patient confidentiality is a frequent basis for a claim or litigation against the facility and its providers.

Why treat patient-related information as confidential? In relation to the biomedical foundational ethical principles, respect for patient confidentiality and privacy evidences respect for patient autonomy. Also, if patients believe that historical information conveyed by them to health care providers will be kept confidential, they are more likely to freely and openly communicate information to their health care providers. That, in turn, facilitates the formulation of accurate diagnoses, which inures to the benefit of patients, providers, the health care organizations and payers, and society. Finally, maintenance of patient confidentiality (absent exceptions discussed in this chapter) is required by state practice acts and implementing regulations, other health-related statutes, and professional codes of ethics. Failure to comply with these directives is a basis for imposition of disciplinary sanctions against providers.

Business Information (Nondisclosure of Proprietary Information)

Health care professionals owe duties of loyalty to entities other than patients under their care. For example, employed health care providers owe a duty of loyalty to their employers. This duty is particularly important in a society like ours, which

> Respect for patient confidentiality and privacy evidences respect for patient autonomy. If patients believe that information conveyed to health care providers will be kept confidential, they are more likely to freely and openly communicate information to their health care providers.

places such a high value on work and particularly on the quality of one's work product. Part of the duty of loyalty owed to one's employer entails the duty (absent exceptions allowed by law and custom) to maintain in confidence proprietary employer information.

It is a breach of ethics (and a violation of civil "tort" law) to misappropriate employer information for employee gain. Consider the following example:

> A rehabilitation clinical manager, who created clinical procedures and quality and risk management manuals for her employer in the course of employment, decides to leave her current position and work for a competing clinic located several blocks away. The clinical manager photocopies the manuals she developed and modifies them only slightly for her new employer. Is this action a violation of law, ethics, or both?

> It is a violation of civil law and of professional and business ethics to expropriate a work product developed by an employee for his or her employer in the course of employment for personal gain or for the gain of a third party. Work products developed incident to an employment relationship are normally the property of the employer, who has paid the employee for the development of such work products.[39]

Other examples of business-related proprietary information for which the employee duty of confidentiality applies include incident reports, peer-review deliberations and findings, and research data. Employers, too, have a reciprocal duty of confidentiality owed to employees and are not free to publicly disseminate, absent waiver or legal mandates, information about employee performance, health status, or discipline.

Permissible and Mandatory Disclosures

The most obvious type of permissible disclosure of otherwise confidential information involves disclosure pursuant to a valid waiver signed by the person(s) whose privacy is affected by the disclosure of information. Typically, patients *expressly* (i.e., explicitly and unambiguously) authorize release of health-related information to third-party payers, health care professional consultants, family members, and others of their choosing. Patients may *impliedly* (i.e., by implication) authorize release of confidential information to other entities, for example, that may include governmental and accreditation reviewers and researchers, among others.

The most obvious type of permissible disclosure of otherwise confidential information involves disclosure pursuant to a valid waiver signed by the person(s) whose privacy is affected by the disclosure of information.

Since, on average, 75 people have access to each patient's confidential health record,[40] patient authorizations for release should clearly state the expected types of professionals and others privileged to invade the patient's privacy and learn confidential information about the patient. Unfortunately, most health-related general releases are woefully inadequate in this regard.

Employees and employers, too, may authorize breaches of confidentiality concerning employee-specific and proprietary information, respectively, through release instruments. For example, a prudent writer of a letter of recommendation for a former employee or student will seek the recommendee's written authorization before disseminating otherwise nonreleasable information about that person.[41]

Mandatory disclosures of personal information occur without regard for permission of the person whose information is disclosed. Most such disclosures are authorized by state or federal law. Such disclosures include, among others, release of information concerning infectious and sexually transmitted diseases to governmental entities, release of information to law enforcement officials upon request or in compliance with reporting statutes, and release of information to third parties pursuant to the federal *Freedom of Information Act* [42] or state freedom of information or open records statutes.

A special case of mandatory release involves the situation in which a patient has communicated a threat of inflicting serious bodily harm or death upon a specified victim. The seminal legal case in this mixed law-ethics area is *Tarasoff v. Regents of the University of California.*[43] In this case a psychotherapist employed by the University of California was treating a mentally ill patient named Poddar. During therapy sessions, Poddar threatened bodily harm against his former girlfriend. The psychotherapist reported the threats to his supervisor, but neither the psychotherapist nor his supervisor reported Poddar's threats to the potential victim or law enforcement authorities.

Poddar carried out his threat and murdered his former girlfriend. Her parents brought legal action against the Regents of the University of California, alleging professional negligence on the part of their agent, the psychotherapist. (The state would be vicariously, or indirectly, liable for the psychotherapist's conduct within the scope of his employment.) In favor of the victim's parents, the California Supreme Court ruled that a psychotherapist owes a legal duty to identifiable third parties threatened by mental patients under their care to warn them of the threats. The court reasoned that, on balance, the duty of confidentiality owed by psychotherapists to patients under their care was outweighed by the court-imposed duty to identifiable third parties to take reasonable steps to warn them of foreseeable serious bodily harm or death at the hands of such patients. This legal duty has ben extended to physicians and other health care professionals in many states.

The duty of confidentiality owed by health care professionals to patients under their care outweighs the court-imposed duty to identifiable third parties to take reasonable steps to warn them of foreseeable serious bodily harm or death at the hands of such patients.

"Routine" disclosures involve releases of personal information not deemed (by legislatures or regulatory agencies) to be confidential to enumerated third parties, made either without a subject's consent or in the absence of an express directive by the subject not to release such information. Examples of routine releases of information include "directory information," (i.e., the presence of a person in a medical facility and the person's condition, place of residence, gender, and age, among other possible information.)[44]

A final area of professional ethical confidentiality involves "discretionary" disclosure of information. The issue of discretionary disclosure of confidential information largely applies to attorneys, who traditionally have been disallowed by professional ethical and state bar rules from disclosing any client confidence, even a client's plan to commit a future crime involving serious bodily harm or death to an identified third party. Some jurisdictions, notably California, are contemplating modifying governing ethics rules to conform with Rule 1.6 of the *Model Rules of Professional Conduct* and allow state-licensed attorneys to electively breach client confidentiality and warn authorities about client plans to commit crimes involving probable serious bodily harm or death to identifiable others.[45]

The concept of discretionary disclosure of confidential information might also apply to a rehabilitation professional who is not protected by a *Tarasoff* law and who discovers, in the course of care delivery, a patient's intent to commit serious bodily harm or death against an identifiable third party. Before breaching patient confidentiality in such cases, health care professionals are urged to consult with facility and/or personal legal counsel for advice.

Ethical Duties of Fidelity and Truthfulness

Closely related to the ethical duty of confidentiality by health care professionals to patients are the duties of fidelity toward and truthfulness in dealings with patients and their significant others. Every health care professional evaluating and treating or otherwise following a patient is a *fiduciary*, or a person in a special position of trust in relation to the patient. Not only are health care professionals obligated under professional ethical standards to act in patients' best interests (i.e., with *beneficence*) but also as fiduciaries, placing the patients' interests above all others—including the financial and other interests of the provider himself or herself.

Regarding truthfulness, it may seem a truism that health care professionals owe patients the duty always to be truthful. Yet there are situations in which health care providers, professional disciplines and organizations, the legal system, and society accept deception of patients and clients as legitimate. One such example involves *therapeutic privilege,* which is addressed in detail in Chapter 3. Other examples of deception in health care clinical practice involve situations less focused

Health care professionals are obligated under professional ethical standards to act in patients' best interests and as fiduciaries, placing the patients' interests above all others.

on beneficence, or patient welfare, and more on provider self-interest. Examples of such deception include the nondisclosure to patients of actual provider conflicts of interest and provider compliance with managed care "gag clauses" in employment or participation contracts that impede full disclosure of treatment-related information to patients.

In her book, *Lying: Moral Choice in Public and Private Life,*[46] Sisela Bok points out that professional ethics codes frequently do not address truthfulness and, even when they do, do not delineate situations in which lying or deception might be justified.[47] One reason this area might not be addressed in detail in health professional codes of ethics is the fact that legitimate justifications for deception of patients, if any exist at all, are relatively rare (e.g., an appropriate application of therapeutic privilege). Also, professional ethics codes do not normally address situation-specific conduct but rather offer broad guidance to professionals under their jurisdiction.

Of the representative rehabilitation codes of ethics that are the focus of this book, only the *Canons of Ethical Conduct* of the American Board for Certification in Orthotics and Prosthetics directly addresses the ethical duty of truthfulness. Canon 3.4 reads:

> All orthotists and prosthetists shall *always* [emphasis added] be truthful and honest to the patient, physician, and public in general.

Gifts

The word *gift* in German means *poison*. Because the areas of patient, referral entity, business associate, vendor, and other sources of gifts to health care providers raise such serious conflict-of-interest ethical concerns, health care providers would do well to remember the German meaning of "gift" when dealing with this issue in most cases.

The *Guide for Professional Conduct* of the American Physical Therapy Association addresses gifts directly. Section 5.4 reads:

> A. Physical therapists shall not accept nor offer gifts or other considerations with obligatory conditions attached.
> B. Physical therapists shall not accept nor offer gifts or other considerations that affect or give an objective appearance of affecting their professional judgment.

In her excellent overview article, "Gift-giving or Influence Peddling: Can You Tell the Difference,"[48] Claudette Finley suggests that patient gifts of *de minimis* monetary value, directed toward an organization, rather than a specific health care provider, are acceptable. Consider the following example:

A neuromuscular rehabilitation patient being discharged after 6 weeks of intensive inpatient care delivers to her occupational therapist a 2-pound box of Godiva chocolates, and expresses her thanks for excellent care rendered. How should the therapist respond?

The occupational therapist should respond by expressing gratitude for the gift on behalf of the entire rehabilitation team, informing the patient that it will be shared with all professional, support, and administrative services team members. In this case, it would probably be unnecessary and might be seen as imprudent to decline the gift altogether.

Summary

Many or most aspects of health professional practice give rise to legal and ethical considerations. Licensure and certification requirements are relatively clear-cut, yet occasionally legal and ethical issues arise, such as professional practice in a state by a provider without prior requisite licensing and/or credentialing. Failure to inquire of state licensure and/or certification entities before practicing one's profession in a state can have profound adverse consequences for providers.

Most health care practice involves unwritten customary practice, not enumerated rules in practice acts. Public and governmental perceptions of intradisciplinary and interdisciplinary health care professional relations affect the status, prestige, and goodwill of health professional disciplines and health care delivery, in general. There is a trend toward multiskilling and cross training in the health and, in particular, the rehabilitation professions, which requires interdisciplinary communication, accommodation, consensus, goodwill, and, where necessary, proposals to modify licensure statutes and regulations and ethical codes of affected health professional disciplines.

In health care delivery, patients have a moral and legal duty to pay fair value for health professional services (absent excusal), while health care providers have multiple ethical and legal duties, including appropriate pricing of services and the maintenance of adequate insurance against potential liability. Health care professionals should consider providing *pro bono publico* service to socioeconomically disadvantaged patients. The problem of patient inability to pay for necessary health services has become more acute under managed care restrictive reimbursement schemes.

The ethical duties of confidentiality, fidelity, and truthfulness owed by health care professionals to patients under their care are paramount and fundamental to patient trust in providers and in the system and compliance with treatment and advice. Providers also owe an ethical duty to employers to safeguard proprietary business information. Confidentiality rules are modified by laws and professional ethical standards involving permissible, mandatory, and discretionary disclosure of information.

The giving or receiving of gifts incident to official health care professional duties raises serious potential issues of conflicts of interest, fraud, lack of independent judgment, and other concerns. Gifts from patients should always be of *de minimis* value and directed toward work teams or organizations, rather than individual providers.

Cases and Questions

1. A physical therapist in private practice sells back- and neck-support devices for a reasonable fee to patients in the clinic. Describe a scenario under which this practice would be unethical.

2. A group of rehabilitation professional co-workers are at lunch in the staff wing of their hospital's cafeteria. An informal discussion ensues concerning the progress of several rehabilitation inpatients. There are no patients or nonhospital employees present; however, several health care professionals from departments other than Rehabilitation Services overhear the conversation. Does this official dialog constitute a breach of professional ethics? Explain.

Suggested Answers for Cases and Questions

1. It would be unethical for the provider to exert undue influence over the patient, such as exaggerating the need for a treatment-related product in order to maximize provider profit.

2. A breach of patient confidentiality has occurred in this scenario, irrespective of the fact that only health professionals heard the information communicated by the rehabilitation team members. The nonrehabilitation team professionals did not have a legitimate "need to know" the confidential information conveyed.

References

1. The Tenth Amendment, United States Constitution, reads: "The powers not delegated to the United States by the Constitution, nor prohibited by it to the States, are reserved to the States respectively, or to the people."

2. *People v. Mari*, 183 NE 858 (NY 1933).

3. *People v. Dennis*, 66 NYS 2d 912 (App Div 1946).

4. Cleverley WO: *Essentials of health care finance*, ed 4, Gaithersburg, Md, 1997, Aspen Publishers, p 283.

5. Sunset update, *Revista OT* 58(6):1, 1993.

6. American Physical Therapy Association: *Guide for professional conduct*, Alexandria, Va, 1997, APTA, Section 3.3A.

7. American Board for Certification in Orthotics and Prosthetics: *Canons of ethical conduct*, Alexandria, Va, 1994, The Board, Section 2.4.

8. Pierson FM: *Principles and techniques of patient care*, Philadelphia, 1994, WB Saunders, pp 20, 25.

9. American Board of Physical Therapy Specialties: *Ceremony for recognition of clinical specialists*, Reno, Nev, 1995, The Board.

10. Hoover S: *Telephonic interview*, Bethesda, Md, (July 10)1997, American Occupational Therapy Association.

11. Association of Rehabilitation Nurses: *Guidelines for evaluating certifications*, Glenview, Ill, 1993, The Association.

12. *Texas disciplinary rules of professional conduct*, Austin, Tex, 1995, Supreme Court of Texas, Rule 7.04b3.

13. *Wilk v. American Medical Association*, 895 F 2d 352, *cert. denied*, 498 US 982 (1990).

14. *The Sherman Act of 1890*, 15 United States Code Section 1.

15. Center for the Health Professions: *Executive summary of the third report of the Pew Health Professions Commission: critical challenges: revitalizing the health professions for the twenty-first century*, San Francisco, (Nov. 17)1995, University of California at San Francisco, p 5.

16. American Board for Certification in Orthotics and Prosthetics: *Canons of ethical conduct*, Alexandria, Va, 1994, The Board, Section 3.10.

17. American Physical Therapy Association: *Guide for professional conduct*, Alexandria, Va, 1997, APTA, Section 3.2.

18. American Occupational Therapy Association: *Occupational therapy code of ethics*, Bethesda, Md, 1994, AOTA, Principles 3E, 3F, 4C.

19. Association of Rehabilitation Nurses: *Position paper: the role of unlicensed assistive personnel in the rehabilitation setting*, Glenview, Ill, 1995, The Association.

20. *Ibid.*

21. Cleverley WO: *Essentials of health care finance*, ed 4, Gaithersburg, Md, 1997, Aspen Publishers, p 222.

22. *Ibid.* pp 53, 61.

23. Lardent EF: Recruitment and retention of volunteer attorneys. In *The resource: a pro bono manual*, Chicago, 1983, American Bar Association, p 7.

24. American Bar Association: *Canons of professional ethics*, Chicago, 1908, ABA.

25. American Bar Association: *Model code of professional responsibility*, Chicago, 1969, ABA.

26. American Bar Association: *Model rules of professional conduct,* Chicago, 1983, ABA.

27. Lardent EF: Pro Bono in the 1990s: the uncertain future of attorney volunteerism. In *Proceedings of the national conference on access to justice in the 1990s,* 1989, Chicago, American Bar Association, p 425.

28. Krieger M: *Professional responsibility class lecture notes,* San Diego, 1983, University of San Diego School of Law.

29. Florida goes halfway in pro bono program, *National Law Journal* 14(27):6, 1992.

30. *US Census Bureau, Statistical Abstract,* ed 110, Washington, DC, 1990, US Government Printing Office.

31. Good Samaritan laws sought for health care workers, *PT Bulletin* 5(23):38, 1990.

32. Relief sought for clinics' malpractice costs, *PT Bulletin* 6(30):5, 1991.

33. Mussman MG, Zawistowich I, Weisman CS: Medical malpractice claims filed by Medicaid and non-Medicaid recipients in Maryland, *JAMA* 265:2992, 1991.

34. Fraiche D: Peer review and the data bank, *Clinical Management* 12(3):14, 1992.

35. Scott RW: *Legal aspects of documenting patient care,* 1994, Gaithersburg, Md, Aspen Publishers, p 10.

36. Ellis J: Clinic provides access to physical therapy for people who are not adequately insured, *PT Bulletin* Sep 19, 1995, p 8.

37. McLaughlin C: PTs donate hands and hearts in reaching out to help the homeless, *Adv Phys Ther* Sep 23, 1996, pp 10, 27.

38. Murphy J: School-based clinic helps uninsured clients, educates students, *Adv Phys Ther* Feb 24, 1997, pp 7, 22.

39. Scott RW: *Promoting legal awareness in physical and occupational therapy,* St Louis, 1997, Mosby, p 248.

40. Siegler M: Confidentiality in medicine—a decrepit concept, *N Engl J Med* 307:1518, 1982.

41. Scott RW: *Promoting legal awareness in physical and occupational therapy,* St Louis, 1997, Mosby, p 214.

42. Scott RW: *Legal aspects of documenting patient care,* 1994, Gaithersburg, Md, Aspen Publishers, p 104.

43. *Tarasoff v. Regents of the University of California,* 17 Cal 3d 425 (1976).

44. Senate Bill 975, 75th Texas Legislature, 1997.

45. McCarthy N: Proposed rule may permit breach of confidentiality, *California Bar Journal* Jul 1997, pp 1, 22.

46. Bok S: *Lying: moral choice in public and private life,* New York, 1989, Vintage Books.

47. *Ibid.* p xvii-xx.

48. Finley C: Gift-giving or influence peddling: can you tell the difference? *J Amer Phys Ther Assoc* 74:143, 1994.

Suggested Readings

Aiken TD, Catalano, JT: *Legal, ethical, and political issues in nursing,* Philadelphia, 1994, FA Davis, ch 3.

American Bar Association: *Canons of professional ethics,* Chicago, 1908, ABA.

American Bar Association: *Model code of professional responsibility,* Chicago, 1969, ABA.

American Bar Association: *Model rules of professional conduct,* Chicago, 1983, ABA.

American Board for Certification in Orthotics and Prosthetics: *Canons of ethical conduct,* Alexandria, Va, 1994, The Board.

American Occupational Therapy Association: *Occupational therapy code of ethics,* Bethesda, Md, 1994, AOTA.

American Occupational Therapy Association: *White paper: occupational therapy and cross-training initiatives,* Bethesda, Md, 1995, AOTA.

American Physical Therapy Association: *Commonalities and differences between the professions of physical therapy and occupational therapy: an American Physical Therapy Association White Paper,* 1994, Alexandria, Va, 1994, APTA.

American Physical Therapy Association: *Directory of certified clinical specialists in physical therapy, 1985-1994,* Alexandria, Va, 1994, APTA.

American Physical Therapy Association: *Guide for conduct of the affiliate member,* Alexandria, Va, 1997, APTA.

American Physical Therapy Association: *Guide for professional conduct,* Alexandria, Va, 1997, APTA.

American Physical Therapy Association: *State licensure reference guide,* Alexandria, Va, 1996, APTA.

Association of Rehabilitation Nurses: *Guidelines for evaluating certifications,* Glenview, Ill, 1993, The Association.

Association of Rehabilitation Nurses: *The role of unlicensed assistive personnel in the rehabilitation setting,* Glenview, Ill, 1995, The Association.

Bailey DM, Schwartzberg SL: *Ethical and legal dilemmas in occupational therapy,* Philadelphia, 1995, FA Davis.

Bok S: *Lying: moral choice in public and private life,* New York, 1989, Vintage Books.

Center for the Health Professions: *Executive summary of the third report of the Pew Health Professions Commission: critical challenges: revitalizing the health professions for the twenty-first century,* San Francisco, (Nov. 17)1995, University of California at San Francisco, p 5.

Ellis J: Clinic provides access to physical therapy for people who are not adequately insured, *PT Bulletin* Sep 19, 1995, p 8.

Finley C: Gift-giving or influence peddling: can you tell the difference? *J Amer Phys Ther Assoc* 74:143, 1994.

Florida goes halfway in pro bono program, *National Law Journal* 14(27):6, 1992.

Fraiche D: Peer review and the data bank, *Clinical Management* 12(3):14, 1992.

Furrow BR, Johnson SH, Jost TS, Schwartz RL: *Health law: cases, materials and problems,* ed 2, 1991, St Paul, Minn, 1991, West Publishing, p 40.

Good Samaritan laws sought for health care workers, *PT Bulletin* 5(23):38, 1990.

Hall MA, Ellman IM: *Health care law and ethics,* St Paul, Minn, 1990, West Publishing.

Lardent EF: Pro bono in the 1990s: the uncertain future of attorney volunteerism. In *Proceedings of the national conference on access to justice in the 1990s,* Chicago, 1989, American Bar Association, p 425.

Lardent EF: Recruitment and retention of volunteer attorneys. In *The resource: a pro bono manual,* Chicago, Ill, 1983, American Bar Association, p 7.

McCarthy N: Proposed rule may permit breach of confidentiality, *California Bar Journal* Jul 1997, pp 1, 22.

McLaughlin C: PTs donate hands and hearts in reaching out to help the homeless, *Adv Phys Ther* Sep 23, 1996, pp 10, 27.

Murphy J: School-based clinic helps uninsured clients, educates students, *Adv Phys Ther* Feb 24, 1997, pp 7, 22.

Mussman MG, Zawistowich I, Weisman CS: Medical malpractice claims filed by Medicaid and non-Medicaid recipients in Maryland, *JAMA* 265:2992, 1991.

Pierson FM: *Principles and techniques of patient care,* Philadelphia, 1994, WB Saunders.

Pozgar GD: *Legal aspects of health care administration,* ed 5, Gaithersburg, Md, 1993, Aspen Publishers.

Purtilo R: *Ethical dimensions in the health professions,* ed 2, Philadelphia, 1993, WB Saunders.

Relief sought for clinics' malpractice costs, *PT Bulletin* 6(30):5, 1991.

Scott RW: *Legal aspects of documenting patient care,* 1994, Gaithersburg, Md, Aspen Publishers.

Siegler M: Confidentiality in medicine—a decrepit concept, *N Engl J Med* 307:1518, 1982.

Tarasoff v. Regents of the University of California, 17 Cal.3d 425, 1976.

US Census Bureau, Statistical Abstract, ed 110, Washington, DC, 1990, US Government Printing Office.

Wilk v. American Medical Association, 895 F 2d 352, *cert. denied,* 498 US 982 (1990).

Nondiscrimination: Considerations of Distributive and Comparative Justice in Health Care Delivery

This chapter addresses patient and provider access issues. Patient access to care issues are discussed first, including the impact of federal and state law on facilitating access to health care services for disabled and geriatric patients. Discrimination issues surrounding HIV and AIDS are explored next, along with relevant legal and professional ethical guidance. Provider access issues are discussed and include employment at will, the Age Discrimination in Employment Act, Title I of the Americans with Disabilities Act, the Civil Rights Acts of 1964 and 1991, and the Family and Medical Leave Act. The chapter concludes with discussion of covenants not to compete in health care employment contracts and "any willing provider" laws protecting providers' rights to participation in managed care health care delivery systems.

•

Patient Access to Health Care Services under Managed Care

Managed care—the private sector analog to public sector health care reform initiatives of the early 1990s—has refocused health care delivery from a unitary quality patient care focus to one that is coprimarily focused on systemic cost containment and quality patient care. Under any system of health care delivery, ethical questions of **distributive** (macro-level) and **comparative** (micro-level) **justice** arise. Policy makers, politicians, providers, and (most importantly) patients are now seriously questioning whether quality patient care is being sacrificed in the name of cost containment under managed care.

Dr. John Ware of the New England Medical Center led a 4-year study of managed care–era health maintenance organizations (HMOs), which found that elder and chronically ill patients with diabetes mellitus, heart disease, hypertension, and depression fared worse in HMOs than under traditional fee-for-service health care plans.[1] Dr. Henry Simmons, MD, MPH, President, National Coalition on Health Care (NCHC), reported at a recent symposium that, under managed care, health care coverage is decreasing and quality patient care is a critical issue. The NCHC favors a cessation of cost shifting of health care to patients and a systemic refocusing on restoring optimal quality patient care.[2]

> Patients are now seriously questioning whether quality patient care is being sacrificed in the name of cost containment under managed care.

Impact of Legal Initiatives on Patient Access to Health Care Services

Recently, states and the federal government have undertaken statutory and regulatory legal initiatives to improve patient access to health care services. A landmark civil rights statute—the Americans With Disabilities Act of 1990[3] (ADA)—empowered 43 million disabled Americans, in part, by affirming their right to access to public facilities (Title II); public accommodations, including privately owned health care facilities (Title III); and telecommunication services (Title IV). The ADA, and particularly its Title I concerning employment rights and duties, is discussed in detail in this chapter.

At least 33 states have enacted patient–protection laws in response to managed care.[4] The federal government has followed the states' lead in this area. One recent federal initiative was the change in the Health Care Financing Administration's (HCFA) Medicare Managed Care appeals process that now provides a 72-hour expedited review of denial of hospitalization.[5] Formerly, HCFA allowed itself 30 to 60 days for all Medicare appeals processing.

AIDS and Other Life-Threatening Illnesses

With over one million Americans having been exposed to the human immunodeficiency virus (HIV),[6] HIV and the resultant acquired immunodeficiency syndrome

(AIDS) are major health problems. Health care professionals unquestionably are under legal and professional ethical duties to treat patients that are HIV-positive and those with AIDS.[7] The ADA recognizes HIV and AIDS as physical disabilities protected under its provisions (i.e., employment [Title I] and access to public and health-related services [Titles II and III]).

None of the representative rehabilitation professional codes of ethics address HIV or AIDS directly in their provisions. All, however, address the symbiotic nature of legal and professional ethical obligations and the requirement to conform professional conduct to the requirements of law.[8,9,10] Canon 3.12 (Illegal Discrimination) of the *Canons of Professional Ethics* of the American Board of Certification in Orthotics and Prosthetics also directly addresses illegal discrimination on the part of providers against patients as follows:

> The orthotist and prosthetist shall not decline to accept a patient on the basis of race, gender, color, religion, or national origin or on any basis [including disability] that would constitute illegal discrimination [parenthetical material added].

Although representative rehabilitation professional ethics codes do not address HIV and AIDS directly, the representative rehabilitation professional associations have issued policy statements expressing the firm commitment of member professionals to treat patients with HIV and AIDS as those with any other potentially life-threatening disease. The AIDS Position Statement of the Association of Rehabilitation Nurses is an example of such a policy statement, and is reprinted in this chapter.[11]

Ethical concerns related to treatment of patients with HIV or AIDS include, among others, confronting one's own prejudices (attitudinal biases), safeguarding patient confidentiality, and protecting third parties who might be at risk of harm because of exposure to the patient's infected bodily fluids.[12] Regarding personal prejudices, health care professionals are obligated by legal and professional ethical standards to sublimate their negative biases, if they cannot overcome them. Similarly, the law and standards of professional ethics disallow the manifestation of negative attitudinal biases against patients (and professional colleagues and others) in the form of (behavioral) prejudices. Patient confidentiality principles remain the same, whether health care professionals are treating patients having AIDS, back pain, or any other condition. (The *Tarasoff* exception to privacy, under which breach of confidentiality is justified to protect identified third parties threatened with serious bodily harm, would apply with equal force to a patient threatening to intentionally infect identified third parties with HIV.) Finally, concerning risk of infection from bodily fluids, the principle of universal precautions requires any health care provider

Health care professionals are obligated by legal and professional ethical standards to sublimate their negative biases. Similarly, the law and standards of professional ethics disallow the manifestation of negative attitudinal biases against patients.

exposed to patient bodily fluids to treat all such patients as potentially infectious and take appropriate self-protective precautions, irrespective of the patient's pathologic condition.

Is there a professional ethical duty to disclose to patients the fact that a health care provider is HIV-positive? Clearly, the incidence of occupational HIV transmission among health care workers is on the increase. From January to June, 1996, the Centers for Disease Control and Prevention (CDC) confirmed 51 documented cases of occupationally acquired HIV infection among health care workers, up from 49 in 1995.[13] Although the representative rehabilitation professional ethics codes are silent on the issue, the CDC recommends only that health care professionals who perform invasive or other exposure-prone procedures on patients be aware of their own HIV status, and that those who are HIV-positive refrain from performing such procedures.[14] Absent a state or federal law requiring otherwise, there is no legal duty to reveal one's HIV status to patients, colleagues, or others. One's HIV status, like one's cancer status, is a private matter—even for clinical health care professionals.

There is no legal duty to reveal the HIV status of health care professionals to patients, colleagues, or others.

Provider Access to Service Delivery

Patients are not the only participants in the managed care arena who face denial of access to health service delivery systems. Health care professionals, too, may face exclusion from participation in health service delivery systems for a variety of reasons—some ethically and legally acceptable, and some not. This section examines some of the key employment law issues having business and professional ethical implications.

Employment "At Will." The vast majority of employees are, as they always have been, employed "at will." Under this traditional common law concept, an employee is free, at any time, to terminate his or her employment with an employer, with or without justification. The reciprocal right rests also with the employer under employment at will. Absent some legally recognized exception, an employer is free, under employment at will, to discharge an employee at any time, with or without just cause.

Employment at will is generally mutually advantageous to employees and employers. Whenever a better employment opportunity arises, an employee knows, under employment at will, that he or she can terminate an existing employment relationship and take advantage of the new opportunity without legal penalty. Similarly, in a time of corporate downsizing, employers can generally adjust the size and composition of their work forces without adverse legal consequences (with due regard to business and professional ethics and social responsibility).

There are, of course, concomitant business and professional ethical implications involving employment at will. For example, when an employed health care professional exercises his or her option, under employment at will, to terminate the employment relationship without due notice to an employer, others besides the employer may suffer adverse consequences. Patients may suffer disruptions in delivery of needed health care professional services, which must be taken into account before such a course of action is undertaken.

There are several recognized exceptions to the concept of employment at will. Obviously, a valid employment contract for a specific term of days, weeks, months, or years is a (contract-based) exception to employment at will. Such a contract must comply with all of the legal requisites for a valid contract, including, among other considerations, a valid offer and acceptance (mutuality of assent), consideration (mutuality of obligation), legal capacity of the parties to contract, legality of the subject matter, and compliance with the state's statute of frauds (requirement for a writing for enforceability of the agreement), as applicable.

Some courts have found that language in employee handbooks, such as a promise not to discharge an employee except for just cause or the promise of "steady employment," imply contractual promises that modify the common law doctrine of employment at will. An employer may be able to disclaim an implied employment contract in an employee handbook by prominently featuring the express disclaimer in the handbook and phrasing it clearly in simple English.[15] Many other employers have chosen to do away with employee handbooks to avoid the possible declaration of an implied employment contract incident to language in the handbook.

Courts have also declared illegal employee discharges based on protected conduct under federal or state statutes. Examples of such wrongful terminations include discharges for "whistle-blowing" (making a good faith report of a suspected violation of law to appropriate authorities); union activities permitted by law; illegal discrimination against racial and ethnic minorities, women, elderly and disabled workers; and the proper filing of workers' compensation and disability claims. Rarely, courts have also declared illegal, as violative of public policy, employee discharges that are deemed fraudulent, malicious, or abusive, such as when a supervisor conspires with co-workers to "create" a case for discharge against an employee.

Similarly, it would constitute wrongful discharge for an employer to terminate an employee who refuses to commit an illegal act. In the rehabilitation setting, an example of such a wrongful discharge might be the situation in a managed care setting in which a licensed or certified health professional is summarily terminated for refusing to allow unqualified extender personnel to carry out clinical duties that cannot legally and/or should not ethically be delegated to them.

Employees are free, at any time, to terminate employment with their employers, with or without justification. The reciprocal right rests also with employers, which are free, under employment at will, to discharge employees at any time, with or without just cause.

Age Discrimination in Employment Act of 1967. The Age Discrimination in Employment Act of 1967 (ADEA),[16] as amended, prohibits employment-related discrimination by private- and public-sector employers of workers age 40 or older (except executives and top policy-making officials). The legal analysis used by courts, administrative agencies, and arbitrators to resolve age discrimination cases under federal law parallels those used in Title VII, Civil Rights Act of 1964 cases. Therefore employment discrimination against older workers is prohibited in recruitment, selection, training, promotion, and conditions of employment.

The ADEA was augmented in 1990 by the Older Workers Benefit Protection Act,[17] which clarified Congress' intent that benefits protection was included in age-related federal antidiscrimination statutory law. The amendment also permits employers to ask dismissed older workers to waive their rights to sue for age discrimination under the ADEA in exchange for compensation.

The Equal Employment Opportunity Commission (EEOC) is the federal agency that administers and enforces the ADEA (and several other federal antidiscrimination laws, discussed below). State statutes and judicial law may afford additional protection to older workers. In 1991 the EEOC and state agencies responsible for protecting older workers' rights processed 27,748 age-discrimination claims.[18]

In recent times, older workers have found it more difficult to prevail in age-discrimination claims and lawsuits brought against employers. At least four federal appellate courts have recently ruled that older workers claiming violations of the ADEA must prove intentional discrimination by their employers and not merely a disproportionate disparate adverse impact of employer actions on older workers.[19] At this writing, the United States Supreme Court has not yet ruled on this matter.

Americans with Disabilities Act of 1990. The ADA[20] was enacted by Congress on July 26, 1990, for the express purpose of "establish[ing] a clear and comprehensive prohibition of discrimination on the basis of disability." [21] This federal statute completed the decades-long effort of Congress, under the Fourteenth Amendment (Due Process and Equal Protection) and under its plenary power to regulate interstate commerce, to prohibit employment discrimination in both the public and private sectors. For the approximately 43 million Americans with physical and mental disabilities, the ADA ensures equal access to public accommodations and services and equal opportunities in employment.

Before the ADA was signed into law, 34 states had already enacted legislation protecting disabled workers against employment-related discrimination. The ADA was modeled after the Rehabilitation Act of 1973,[22] which prohibits disability-related employment discrimination in federal executive agencies and by the approximately 50 percent of private sector businesses that contract with the federal government.

Approximately 43 million Americans with physical and mental disabilities are ensured equal access to public accommodations and services and equal opportunities in employment.

The ADA has five sections, or "titles," that protect the rights of people with disabilities. Title I (discussed in greater detail in this chapter) protects against disability-related employment discrimination. Title II ensures equal access for the disabled to public services (i.e., all activities of state and local governments), including public transportation services. Title III ensures equal access for the disabled to public accommodations, including all private businesses and services (except for some private clubs and all religious organizations, including places of worship[23]). Title III includes, under its jurisdiction, private health care facilities. Title IV provides for equal access by disabled patrons to telecommunications services. Title V is a miscellaneous section addressing, among other considerations, the relationship of the ADA to other federal statutes, key definitions, and an affirmation that the states cannot claim (Eleventh Amendment) immunity from the requirements of the ADA.

Title I became effective on July 26, 1992, for businesses employing 25 or more people, and on July 26, 1994, for businesses with 15 or more employees. Title I covers private and public employers and employment agencies and union organizations.

Title I of the ADA prohibits employment discrimination by employers against employees and job applicants who are qualified to perform the essential functions of their jobs. This prohibition against employment discrimination is all-encompassing, applying to recruitment, selection, training, benefits, promotion, discipline, and retention. The ADA does not, however, establish a quota system for hiring or retaining disabled workers.

If a job candidate with a disability is legitimately found to be unable to perform the essential functions of a position, that person may be rejected as a candidate for employment for that position. The legal burden of challenging such a decision rests with the rejected candidate, who must prove that he or she is the best-qualified person for the position. Qualification standards also require that a candidate not pose a "direct threat" to others in the workplace, that is, "a significant risk to the health or safety of others that cannot be eliminated by reasonable accommodation."[24]

Title I includes several key definitions. **Disability** is defined in one of three ways[25] as an employee or job applicant who:

- Has a physical or mental impairment that substantially limits one or more major life activities
- Has a record of such an impairment
- Is regarded as having such an impairment

Major life activities include all of the important activities of daily living already well-known to rehabilitation professionals, including the ability to see and hear, speech, cardiorespiratory functions, ambulation, self-care, the performance of manual tasks, and formal and informal learning activities, among others.[26]

Precisely which functions are "essential" for any given job is a matter of business judgment for employers.[27] Prudent liability risk management, adherence of

> The ADA prohibits employment discrimination by employers against employees and job applicants who are qualified to perform the essential functions of their jobs; this prohibition applies to recruitment, selection, training, benefits, promotion, discipline, and retention.

business ethical responsibilities, and fundamental fairness require, however, that standards in job descriptions and delineation of essential functions for positions be clear, justifiable, and in writing. Business decisions regarding the labeling of job tasks as "essential functions" should be reviewed by legal counsel before implementation.

A **qualified individual with a disability** is a job applicant or employee who can perform essential job functions, with or without reasonable accommodation.[28] **Reasonable accommodation** is defined by the EEOC[29] as:

> [A]ny change or adjustment to a job or work environment that permits a qualified applicant or employee with a disability to participate in the job application process, to perform the essential functions of a job, or to enjoy benefits and privileges of employment equal to those enjoyed by employees without disabilities...and may include:
> - Acquiring or modifying equipment or devices
> - Job restructuring
> - Part-time or modified work schedules
> - Reassignment to a vacant position
> - Adjusting or modifying examinations, training materials, or policies
> - Providing readers and interpreters
> - Making the workplace readily accessible to and usable by people with disabilities

Reasonable accommodation must be carried out upon request of an applicant or employee (or by the employer if a disability is obvious), unless the employer can prove that to do so would amount to an undue hardship. **Undue hardship** is defined as a situation in which accommodation is excused because to do so would be unduly burdensome (excessively disruptive, costly, or difficult to implement), or would fundamentally alter the very nature of the employer's business operations.[30] The accommodation provided need not be one specifically requested by a disabled applicant or employee but one that enables the applicant or employee to perform the essential functions of his or her job. The applicant or employee can be asked to contribute to funding the accommodation if its cost amounts to an undue hardship for the employer.[31]

The ADA does not require that employers hire or promote anyone but the "best qualified"; however, the law mandates that disabled applicants and employees be afforded equal consideration in the selection process. Excluded from the statutory definition of **disabled** are the following:
- Current illegal drug users and abusers of alcohol
- Compulsive gamblers, kleptomaniacs, and pyromaniacs
- Pedophiles, exhibitionists, and voyeurs
- Homosexuals and bisexuals

Employers are not required to hire or promote anyone but the "best qualified"; however, the law mandates that disabled applicants and employees be afforded equal consideration in the selection process.

- Persons with gender identification and miscellaneous sexual behavior disorders (including transsexualism and transvestism)[32]

Employers must continuously review their hiring, promotion, training, and benefits programs to ensure compliance with the ADA. They must especially ensure that, during the hiring process, prospective employees are judged on their abilities, not disabilities, and that candidates and current employees are made aware of their ADA rights (through posting of federal antiemployment-discrimination requirements in a prominent place[33]).

Regarding preemployment inquiries and screening tests, the following rules apply. It is unlawful to inquire about applicants' disabilities and to require preoffer medical examinations. Preoffer drug screening tests, however, are permissible actions by management, as are nonmedical-related physical agility and psychological tests.

Once a conditional offer has been extended to an applicant, it is permissible to carry out a job-related medical examination, if such an examination is universally given to all similarly situated conditional offerees. A final offer of employment may lawfully be conditioned on the results of such an examination.

According to final EEOC regulations on preemployment questions released in October 1995, it is permissible for an employer to inquire about an applicant's ability to perform specific tasks, including requiring a demonstration of job skills, so long as such an inquiry is made of all applicants. Although it is generally unlawful to inquire about reasonable accommodation(s) during preoffer interviews, the EEOC sanctions such inquiries when:

- Employer reasonably believes that reasonable accommodation might be required for a job, because the applicant displays an obvious disability, such as blindness or paralysis
- Applicant voluntarily discloses an unidentified disability, and the employer reasonably believes that accommodation might be required
- Applicant requests accommodation

The EEOC establishes rules and regulations that interpret the ADA and enforces the mandates of the Act. Although there were a relatively small number of claims of disability-related job discrimination lodged by complainants with the EEOC during 1992 (approximately 400 per month), the number of complaints grew to 1600 per month by March 1993.[34] By the end of 1994, the EEOC had processed over 30,000 claims. The specific impairment most often cited in complaints was back-pain syndrome (20 percent), followed by neurological impairment (12 percent), and emotional and psychiatric impairment (11 percent).[35] A quarter of all ADA complaints lodged with the EEOC relate to the alleged failure on the part of employers to provide appropriate reasonable accommodation for disabled applicants and employees.[36]

Litigation over the scope of duty on the part of employers to provide reasonable accommodation to disabled workers has helped clarify the mandates of

107

the ADA. For example, courts have ruled in favor of employees, requiring a teacher's aide for a teacher with physical and mental limitations after an automobile accident,[37] reasonable alternatives for an employee unable to drive (an "essential function") because of terminal cancer,[38] lifting restrictions for a nurse with lower back dysfunction,[39] home-based work for a clerical employee with multiple sclerosis,[40] health professional licensure boards to consider mental illness and a history of drug or alcohol abuse as disabilities covered under the ADA,[41] and law examining boards to make requested special accommodations for attorney applicants with dyslexia,[42] among other required accommodations. Courts have also ruled in favor of employers, holding that extensive workplace redesign required to accommodate a paraplegic employee constitutes excessive cost and undue hardship,[43] accommodation short of a total workplace smoking ban for an asthmatic employee is acceptable,[44] and many mental disability claims based on nonspecific or subjective diagnoses are invalid (in some instances, in opposition to the EEOC's position),[45] among other decisions in favor of the employer.

Courts are divided, in reasonable accommodation ADA litigation cases, over whether the employee or the employer bears the legal burden of proof in the case. Some courts take a middle ground, first requiring a disabled employee to establish that he or she can perform the essential functions of a particular job (with or without accommodation) and then shifting the burden of proof to the employer to establish why the employer should be excused from providing accommodation.[46]

Despite the substantial number of administrative and litigation cases involving the ADA, employers should not be fearful of the ADA. In addition to reflecting the highest standards of business ethics and reinforcing a business' social responsibility to recruit, hire, train and develop, retain, and promote workers with disabilities, the ADA makes good business sense. Total public support of a person who has a disability averages 1 million dollars over the person's lifetime, whereas employment of that person results in a net gain to public coffers of $65,000 in taxes paid. Studies and experience show that people with disabilities want to work and perform their work very well, relative to the total work force. One recent study concluded that persons with severe physical or mental disabilities or both can be successful in the workplace through supported employment.[47]

Employers who are strongly committed to the principles of the ADA also benefit from an enhanced public image and increased goodwill. Employers should not take a defensive approach to compliance with the ADA because, as has been the case with health care malpractice prevention, a defensive posture only serves to increase the likelihood of litigation.

Despite the call from some legislators in the current Congress for ADA reform, based in part on the financial burden of compliance,[48] the ADA remains a "linchpin" for employment and civil rights, crucial to the prestige and maintenance of

Public support of a person who has a disability averages 1 million dollars over the person's lifetime, whereas employment results in a net gain of $65,000 in taxes paid. Studies and experience show that people with disabilities want to work and perform their work very well, relative to the total work force.

the United States as a world leader. Rehabilitation professionals have a unique opportunity to serve as consultants to both employers (to help them meet their legal responsibilities) and to employees (to assist them in exercising their rights and rehabilitation and vocational potential).

Civil Rights Acts of 1964 and 1991. The most important, or at least most pervasive, federal statute addressing employment discrimination and civil rights is Title VII of the Civil Rights Act of 1964.[49] This law was critically important for the full integration of racial and other minorities into the American work force, yet its passage was stalled for years in the United States Senate by repeated filibusters.

President John F. Kennedy, Attorney General Robert Kennedy, and congressional Democratic leaders grounded the statute in Congress' plenary power to regulate interstate commerce,[50] rather than in constitutional due process or equal protection under law, believing this was the only way the law could survive a legal challenge by noncompliant private sector businesses. The legal premise justifying enactment of the Civil Rights Act of 1964 was that discrimination of minorities—especially African Americans—by business entities had an immeasurable adverse impact on interstate commerce, and, consequently, Congress was empowered to remedy this situation by means of a federal nondiscrimination mandate to all public and private business entities.

Title VII specifically prohibits discrimination against job applicants and employees on the basis of race or ethnicity, gender (as of 1972), religion, and national origin, at all stages along the continuum of employment processes. The groups enumerated in Title VII are referred to in case and administrative law as "protected classes." Specifically, Title VII states in pertinent part that:

It shall be an unlawful employment practice for an employer:

1. To fail or refuse to hire or to discharge any individual, or otherwise to discriminate against any individual with respect to his [or her] compensation, terms, conditions, or privileges of employment, because of such individual's race, color, religion, sex, or national origin;

2. To limit, segregate, or classify...employees or applicants for employment in any way that would deprive any individual of employment opportunities or otherwise adversely affect his [or her] status as an employee, because of such individual's race, color, religion, sex, or national origin.[51]

Title VII applies to all private sector businesses with 15 or more employees; labor unions; and federal, state, and local governmental entities. Title VII is administered and enforced by the EEOC. States are free to provide additional constitutional, statutory, judicial, and administrative protections to their citizens, over and above that provided by federal law. Forty-one states, the District of Columbia, and Puerto Rico all have statutes similar to Title VII.[52]

Employers are required by EEOC regulations to create, submit for review, and maintain records that evidence compliance with Title VII. For reporting purposes, race (ethnicity) is divided into five classifications: white (non-Hispanic), black, Hispanic, Asian or Pacific Islander, and American Indian or Alaskan native.[53]

Title VII expressly permits employment discrimination against protected classes of persons on the basis of bona fide occupational qualifications (BFOQs).[54] A BFOQ must be based on legitimate business necessity, that is, it must be reasonably necessary for the normal operation of a particular business. BFOQs are allowed for gender, religion, and national origin (and age under the ADEA) classifications, provided that employers can establish business necessity. (BFOQs based on race violate public policy and are generally disallowed.) An example of a legitimate gender-based BFOQ is the requirement, based on social mores, that dressing room attendants be the same gender as patrons. An example of a legitimate religion-based BFOQ is the requirement that a parish priest be Catholic.

Title VII prohibits both intentional and unintentional employment discrimination. Intentional employment discrimination is referred to as "disparate treatment," whereas other employment practices, though they appear to be protected class–neutral on their face, have a particular adverse or "disparate impact" on the employment rights of protected class members.

The Civil Rights Act of 1991[55] was enacted to clarify congressional intent regarding employment discrimination after the United States Supreme Court reportedly "weakened the scope and effectiveness of federal civil rights protections"[56] in its 1989 decision in *Wards Cove Packing Co. v. Atonio.*[57] The provisions of this federal statute affect the Civil Rights Act of 1964 and the Rehabilitation Act of 1973.

The Civil Rights Act of 1991 invalidates the Supreme Court's holding in *Wards Cove,* in part, by reshifting part of the burden of proof in "disparate impact" employment discrimination cases from plaintiffs to employers, who must once again prove business necessity for any business practice that is proven (by a plaintiff) to have a "disparate impact" on a Title VII–protected class.

The Civil Rights Act of 1991 also permits, for the first time, not only the equitable remedies of reinstatement, back pay (with interest), and restoration of seniority for proven employment discrimination, but it also allows compensatory and punitive damages for intentional discrimination under Title VII or the ADA. Title VII and ADA plaintiffs have the right, for the first time, to request a jury trial for determination of money damages. Money damages are graduated according to company size and are capped at $300,000.[58]

Prohibited for the first time under the Civil Rights Act of 1991 is the process of "race norming," under which raw scores on preemployment tests were sometimes scaled differently for racial and ethnic minority applicants as a form of affirmative action. The law also protects United States citizens who are employed outside of

---

The Civil Rights Act of 1991 permits not only the equitable remedies of reinstatement, back pay (with interest), and restoration of seniority for proven employment discrimination, but it also allows compensatory and punitive damages for intentional discrimination.

the United States from employment discrimination by United States firms. (An exception to this extraterritorial application of Title VII is that firms are allowed to comply with local foreign customs in their employment practices.)

Family and Medical Leave Act of 1993. The Family and Medical Leave Act of 1993 (FMLA)[59] was signed into law by President Clinton just after his inauguration and became effective on February 5, 1993. The FMLA requires covered employers to provide up to 12 weeks of unpaid, job- and benefit-protected leave per year to eligible employees for childbirth, adoption, and personal and family medical illnesses. About 45 million workers in the United States are eligible to take advantage of the FMLA.[60]

Employees eligible for FMLA protection are those who have worked for at least 1250 hours during the previous 12 months at a location in which their employer has 50 or more employees located within a 75-mile radius. Under Department of Labor administrative rules, which became effective in April 1995, covered illnesses under the FMLA include those conditions that incapacitate an employee or family member (spouse, child, or parent) for at least 3 days, require consultation with a health care professional, and are treated with prescription medications.[61]

Under the administrative rules implementing the FMLA, an employee on FMLA leave of absence for personal illness is not required to accept an employer's offer of "light duty" or other reasonable accommodation.[62] This rule is seemingly inconsistent with the ADA and probably results in significant confusion on the part of human resource managers who must co-administer the FMLA and the ADA for their companies. Interagency coordination and reconciliation of this inconsistency, on the part of the Department of Labor and EEOC, is needed.

Although eligible employees must provide a 30-day advance notice of covered leave whenever feasible, employers fear abuses and an adverse effect on productivity.[63] Employers may require the production of a medical certificate of illness and even a second opinion regarding a claimed covered illness (at the employer's expense). Employer retaliation against an employee invoking the protection of the FMLA is prohibited. The law is enforced by the United States Department of Labor. Consider the following example:

> A rehabilitation aide working for a health care organization covered by the FMLA requests FMLA leave to care for her spouse, who has diabetes mellitus and is recovering from a left below-knee amputation. The employer wants to discharge this employee because of her efforts to unionize eligible rehabilitation staff. The employer authorizes FMLA leave for only 1 week, hoping that the employee will quit. Discuss the legal and ethical issues raised by the scenario.

About 45 million employees in the United States are eligible to take advantage of the provisions of the Family and Medical Leave Act.

111

The employer is not free to unilaterally and arbitrarily set the time period for FMLA leave. It is a matter for joint decision making by the employee (with input from her spouse's physicians and other rehabilitation providers) and the employer, with employee substantiation of need, as required. The employer in this case has violated the FMLA and labor laws, which disallow employer retaliation for legitimate union activities, and has breached business ethics by arbitrarily setting a short FMLA leave period to induce the employee to resign her position.

Restrictive Covenants in Employment Contracts

Restrictive covenants in employment contracts limit the ability of parties to act without restraint in specified ways. In health care contracts, the principal types of restrictive covenants affecting employees are the nonsolicitation provision and the covenant not to compete. A nonsolicitation clause in an employment contract prevents a former professional employee from marketing his or her professional services to the employer's existing clients after termination of the employment relationship. A covenant not to compete is a contractual general promise made by an employee not to compete directly with a former employer.

A covenant not to compete is, in essence, a restraint on trade, which is generally considered to be against public policy. For that reason, a few states prohibit it altogether in employment contracts.[64] Most states, however, allow the covenant not to compete in employment contracts as a means to protect an employer's legitimate business interests.[65]

A covenant not to compete in an employment contract must meet four criteria to be valid and enforceable:

- It must be supported by consideration, that is, the covenant not to compete must have been made as part of a bargained-for exchange, and value must have been given by the employer in exchange for the employee's promise not to compete.
- A covenant not to compete must be reasonable in three areas[66]:
  - ▲ Geographic area of practice restriction
  - ▲ Specific practice restrictions
  - ▲ Time

In a recent Ohio court case, a not-to-compete clause in an employment contract between a physical therapist and a health care organization purportedly disallowed the physical therapist from carrying out professional services (after employment was terminated) with any patients who were former customers of the organization. The appellate court found the clause ambiguous and *reformed* the contract to modify the covenant not to compete so as *only* to disallow the physical therapist from directly competing for contracts (in the geographic area) with the organization after termination of employment.[67]

"Any Willing Provider" Laws

"Any willing provider" laws are state laws designed to safeguard the rights of licensed and certified health care professionals to freely practice their professions and to participate in health care delivery services under managed care. Generally, under these laws, all qualified providers who are willing to participate in managed care health delivery services and who are able to meet the reasonable inclusion standards of managed care organizations, insurers, or other payers, must be included in provider networks. Absent the existence of "any willing provider" laws in a state, managed care organizations may contract exclusively with select health care providers and groups for service delivery and exclude all others from participation. As of 1995, 25 states have enacted "any willing provider" laws. In 17 of these states, the protection applies only to pharmacists, who are deemed most likely to be adversely affected by exclusive provider arrangements under managed care.[68]

General versus Limited-Scope Practice Settings: the Issue of Patient Abandonment

Rehabilitation professionals whose clinical practices encompass a limited scope of practice (such as exclusively hand rehabilitation or sports-related orthotics, prosthetics, or therapy) are advised to clearly communicate the fact of their limited scope of practice to patients about to come under their care. By doing so, limited-scope practice providers ensure that patients understand the limited legal duty owed by such providers. Such disclosure also demonstrates respect for patient autonomy in choosing a provider for care. It may prevent a claim of patient abandonment in the event that a patient under such circumstances requests additional services not provided by the limited-scope providers and is therefore denied care.

Summary

Access to health care service delivery for patients and health care professionals has become more complicated under managed care. For patients, the problem of under-delivery of needed health care services—often called *reverse fraud and abuse*—affects their health and well-being. For health care professionals, the denial of the opportunity to participate in managed care service networks in many cases equates to the inability to practice their professions.

State legislatures and Congress have recently enacted legislation protecting patients' and providers' right of access to health care service delivery systems. Included among patient protective measures are the ADA (Titles II and III) and regulatory initiatives designed to give Medicare patients broader appeal rights for denial of care. Providers benefit from the ADA (Title I), the Civil Rights Acts of 1964 and 1991, the FMLA, and "any willing provider" laws. Providers should consult with personal legal counsel before signing employment contracts containing covenants not to compete.

Legislation alone will not ensure patient and provider access to health care delivery service systems. Patients, health care professionals, health policy makers, and politicians must work jointly to resolve dilemmas involving patient and provider access to health care services. Providers and health care organizations must also adhere to the highest standards of professional ethics and, where compatible with professional ethics, of business ethics, to provide optimal quality care to those patients under their care.

Cases and Questions

1. A physical therapist declines to perform wound care procedures on patients, citing "personal reasons," without stating a specific reason to her supervisor. The supervisor suspects that the therapist may be hiding that she is HIV-positive. Can the supervisor compel the therapist to reveal the reason for declining to carry out wound care activities on patients?

2. A physical therapist–owned home health agency, XYZ Company, offers to contract with A, a new graduate physical therapist, for employment. The written employment contract contains XYZ Company's standard covenant not to compete, which reads:

   A and XYZ Company agree that, in the event of termination of employment by A with XYZ Company, A will not: (1) practice home health physical therapy in the state of Pennsylvania, (2) for a period of 5 years. A asks to take the contract with her for review by her and her legal counsel. The President of XYZ Company refuses, and demands that A either sign the contract in XYZ Company's office or forego the employment opportunity with XYZ Company. What ethical and legal concerns, if any, are raised by this scenario?

Suggested Answers for Cases and Questions

1. The physical therapist cannot be compelled to disclose her condition but may have to justify her declination of duties by having her personal physician verify that she has a medical condition that necessitates that she not carry out invasive procedures.

114

continued

Suggested Answers for Cases and Questions—cont'd

2. The covenant not to compete in this scenario is unreasonable, in terms of time, practice restrictions, and geographic scope of coverage. The employer and prospective employee should bargain in good faith over the terms of any required covenant not to compete in their employment contract.

References

1. Anders G: Quality of care for poor and elderly at HMOs is questioned in new study, *Wall Street Journal* B6, (Oct. 2)1996.

2. Ketter P: Experts revisit health care reform: examine quality of care, outcomes issues, *PT Bulletin* Jul 11, 1997, pp 8-9.

3. The Americans With Disabilities Act of 1990, 42 United States Code Sections 12101-12213.

4. Managed care consumer protection laws enacted in more than 30 states, *PT Bulletin* pp 1, 12, Aug 2, 1996.

5. Mayo Pi-Yi: Medicare basics. In *University of Texas Elder Law Conference,* Austin, Tex, 1997, University of Texas School of Law, pp 24-25.

6. Association of Rehabilitation Nurses: *AIDS position statement,* Glenview, Ill, 1986, The Association.

7. Gibeaut J: Filling a need, *ABA Journal* 83(7):48, 1997.

8. American Board of Certification in Orthotics and Prosthetics: *Canons of professional ethics,* Alexandria, Va, 1994, ABC Canon 3.8 (Compliance with Laws and Regulations).

9. American Physical Therapy Association: *Guide for professional conduct,* Alexandria, Va, 1997, APTA Section 2.1 (Professional Practice).

10. American Occupational Therapy Association: *Occupational therapy code of ethics,* Bethesda, Md, 1994, AOTA Principle 4A.

11. See note 6.

12. Brecker LR: Physical therapists face ethical dilemmas in treating patients with HIV and AIDS, *Advance for Physical Therapists* 22-23:58, 1993.

13. *Occupational HIV transmission up in 1996,* Oct 25, 1996, Reuters.

14. Scheerhorn M: Disclosure of health care workers with HIV or AIDS, *Nursing Management* 26(10):48, 1995.

15. Furey MK, Ohnegian SA: Employee handbooks may be implied contracts, *National Law Journal* B12, Oct 24, 1994.

16. The Age Discrimination in Employment Act of 1967, 29 United States Code Sections 621-634.

17. The Older Workers Benefit Protection Act of 1990, 29 United States Code Section 623.

18. Perry PM: Don't get sued for age discrimination, *Law Practice Management* May/Jun, 1995.

19. McMorris FA: Age-bias suits may become harder to prove, *Wall Street Journal* B1, Feb 20, 1997.

20. See note 3.

21. Preamble: The Americans with Disabilities Act of 1990, Public Law 101-336.

22. The Rehabilitation Act of 1973, 29 United States Code Sections 794a.

23. 42 United State Code Section 12187.

24. 42 United States Code Section 12111.

25. 42 United States Code Section 12102.

26. Equal Employment Opportunity Commission: *The Americans with Disabilities Act: your responsibilities as an employer,* Washington, DC, 1991, EEOC Publication No. EEOC-BK-17, p 2.

27. 42 United States Code Section 12111.

28. *Ibid.*

29. Equal Employment Opportunity Commission: *The Americans with Disabilities Act: your responsibilities as an employer,* Washington, DC, 1991, EEOC Publication No. EEOC-BK-17, p 4.

30. *Ibid,* pp 5-6; 42 United States Code Sections 12111.

31. Equal Employment Opportunity Commission: *The Americans with Disabilities Act: your responsibilities as an employer,* Washington, DC, 1991, EEOC Publication No. EEOC-BK-17, p 6.

32. 42 United States Code Sections 12114, 12211.

33. Equal Employment Opportunity Commission: *The Americans with Disabilities Act: your responsibilities as an employer,* Washington, DC, 1991, EEOC Publication No. EEOC-BK-17, p 15.

34. Disability cases rise, *Wall Street Journal,* B10, May 6, 1993.

35. Backlash with ADA emerging, education needed, *PT Bulletin* 15, Feb 24, 1995.

36. Mirone JA: Reasonable accommodation in disability law, *PT: the magazine of physical therapy* 3(3):68, 1995.

37. Borkowski v. Valley Central District, 63 F.2d 131 (2d, ca 1995).

38. EEOC v. AIC Security Investigations, Ltd, 820 F. Supp. 1060 (ND Ill, 1993).

39. Tuck v. HCA Health Services of Tennessee, Inc, 7 F.3d 465 (6th, ca 1993).

40. Langan v. Department of Health and Human Services, 959 F.2d 1053 (Washington, DC, ca 1992).

41. ADA limits licensure boards, *PT Bulletin* 13, Jul 11, 1997.

42. Aspiring lawyer with dyslexia gets test access, *Wall Street Journal* B1-B2, Jul 18, 1997.

43. Vande Zande v. Wisconsin Department of Administration, 44 F.3d 538 (7th, ca 1995).

44. Harmer v. Virginia Electric & Power Company, 831 F. Supp. 1300 (ED Vir, 1993).

45. Courts reject many mental-disability claims, *Wall Street Journal* B1, B6, Jul 22, 1997.

46. Phelan G: Reasonable accommodation: linchpin of ADA liability, *Trial* pp 40-44, at 44, Feb 1996. In this excellent overview article, the author describes many additional reasonable accommodation ADA cases. For additional reasonable accommodation ADA cases, see Mirone JA, note 32.

47. Wehman P, Revell W, Kregel J, et al: Supported employment: an alternative model for vocational rehabilitation of persons with severe neurological, psychiatric, or physical disability, *Arch Phys Med Rehabil* 72(2):101, 1991.

48. States, cities stagger under financial burden of disabilities law, *PT Bulletin* pp 36-37, Dec 15, 1993.

49. The Civil Rights Act of 1964, Title VII, 42 United States Code Section 2000e-2000e-17.

50. United States Constitution, Article I, Section 8.

51. The Civil Rights Act of 1964, Title VII, Section 703(a).

52. Cherrington DJ: *The management of human resources,* ed 4, Englewood Cliffs, NJ, 1995, Prentice-Hall, p 95.

53. 29 Code of Federal Regulations Sections 1602.20(b), 1607.4(B), 1993.

54. The Civil Rights Act of 1964, Title VII, Section 703(e).

55. The Civil Rights Act of 1991, Public Law 102-166, 105 Stat. 071, 42 United States Code Sections 1981a and 2000e.

56. 42 United States Code 1981 note.

57. Wards Cove Packing Co. v. Atonio, 490 U.S. 642 (1989).

58. Davidson MJ: The Civil Rights Act of 1991, *Army Lawyer* 3-11 at 3-4, Mar 1992,

59. The Family and Medical Leave Act of 1993, 29 United States Code Section 2601-2654.

60. Lublin JS: Family-leave law can be excuse for a day off, *Wall Street Journal* B1, B10, Jul 7, 1995.

61. *Ibid*, at B1.

62. Young RS: Managing medical leaves of absence, *HR Magazine* 23-30, Aug 1995.

63. *Ibid*, citing Survey of 123 Fortune 500 companies by Labor Policy Association, Washington, DC.

64. Lewis K: Physical therapy contracts, *Clinical Management* 12(6):14, 1992. Most states that prohibit employment-related covenants not to compete permit such contractual provisions involving the sale of an ongoing business to another professional, in order to protect the "goodwill" value of the business being sold.

65. Wallen E: A restrictive covenant can lessen practice's risk of losing patients, *Physicians Financial News* 26, May 1991.

66. Freed C, Martinez WL: Non-compete covenant has to be reasonable, *San Antonio Medical Gazette* 8, Jun 9-15, 1993.

67. Concept Rehab, Inc. v. Short, *Lawyers Weekly*, No. 106-083-97 (6th Ohio District Court of Appeals, 1997).

Suggested Readings

The Age Discrimination in Employment Act of 1967, 29 United States Code Sections 621-634.

The Americans With Disabilities Act of 1990, 42 United States Code Sections 12101-12213.

Anders G: Quality of care for poor and elderly at HMOs is questioned in new study, *Wall Street Journal* B6, (Oct. 2)1996.

Association of Rehabilitation Nurses: *AIDS position statement,* Glenview, Ill, 1986, The Association.

Brecker LR: Physical therapists face ethical dilemmas in treating patients with HIV and AIDS, *Advance for Physical Therapists* 22-23:58, 1993.

Cherrington DJ: *The management of human resources,* ed 4, Englewood Cliffs, NJ, 1995, Prentice-Hall, p 95.

The Civil Rights Act of 1964, Title VII, 42 United States Code Section 2000e-2000e-17.

The Civil Rights Act of 1991, 42 United States Code Sections 1981a and 2000e.

Equal Employment Opportunity Commission: *The Americans with Disabilities Act: your responsibilities as an employer,* Washington, DC, 1991, EEOC Publication No. EEOC-BK-17.

The Family and Medical Leave Act of 1993, 29 United States Code Section 2601-2654.

Furey MK, Ohnegian SA: Employee handbooks may be implied contracts, *National Law Journal* B12, Oct 24, 1994.

Gibeaut J: Filling a need, *ABA Journal* 83(7):48, 1997.

Goldfein RB, Hanssens C: Protecting HIV-positive workers: whose ADA is it anyway? *Trial* 26-31, Feb, 1996.

Ketter P: Experts revisit health care reform: examine quality of care, outcomes issues, *PT Bulletin* Jul 11, 1997, pp 8-9.

Lewis K: Physical therapy contracts, *Clinical Management* 12(6):14, 1992.

Managed care consumer protection laws enacted in more than 30 states, *PT Bulletin* pp 1, 12, Aug 2, 1996.

McMorris FA: Age-bias suits may become harder to prove, *Wall Street Journal* B1, Feb 20, 1997.

Perry PM: Don't get sued for age discrimination, *Law Practice Management* May/Jun, 1995.

The Rehabilitation Act of 1973, 29 United States Code Sections 794a.

Scheerhorn M: Disclosure of health care workers with HIV or AIDS, *Nursing Management* 26(10):48, 1995.

Professional Business Arrangements and Considerations

This chapter addresses some of the salient health professional business-related ethical concerns affecting clinical practice. These issues include referral of patients for profit, actual and perceived conflicts of interest, ethical concerns in business contracts, professional advertising, fraud and abuse, and impaired providers. The chapter includes several hypothetical case examples illustrating ethical problems affecting professional practice, in addition to the customary end-of-chapter cases and questions.

•

Although health care service delivery is normally a commercial business (even when "not-for-profit"), it is not just another business enterprise. Health care service delivery involves caring for patients and clients who are injured or ill and therefore uniquely vulnerable to exploitation. For that reason, in part, strict codes of professional ethics govern the official conduct of licensed and certified health care professionals and, for many disciplines, their assistants and extender personnel as well. In fact, the professional ethical standards governing members of health care disciplines are at least as strict as, and quite similar to, the ethical rules governing the official conduct of attorneys, who manage clients' personal, business, and financial affairs and, in criminal law venues, defend clients against the possible loss of life and liberty.

Because of this special status of health care service delivery in society and under law, it is inaccurate, if not inappropriate, to refer to the business of health care as an *industry*. Health care providers, clinical managers, administrators, educators, leaders of professional associations and licensure and certification entities, and relevant others, are strongly encouraged to refocus their clients and other customers and users of the health care delivery system—internal and external—on the special nature and status of health care and to challenge the use of the phrase, the *health care industry*, whenever it is used. (One never hears the phrase, the *legal industry* when referring to the legal profession. The same should apply with equal force to health care professions and service.)

Practice Arrangements and Affiliations

Health professional ethical and related legal standards permit a wide range of variegated health professional practice arrangements involving participants from multiple disciplines. Although group-practice arrangements may simply involve a number of health professionals from different disciplines carrying out independent practices in a common *situs*—(i.e., **multidisciplinary** practice), rehabilitation practice involves professionals and support personnel from multiple disciplines working in concert toward common goals for patients and is an example of **interdisciplinary** (group) practice.

There are a number of professional ethical problems, issues, and dilemmas involved in the business of health care delivery, whether in group or individual practice. Many, if not most, of these concerns center on whose interests predominate—those of patients or those of provider(s) and others. One such issue (discussed in detail in Chapter 3) involves the decision of whether to reveal to patients during informed consent disclosure the fact that their health care providers may be paid by an employing entity, in whole or in part, on the basis of minimizing health care delivery and related costs. Others involve self-referral and solicitation or acceptance of patient referrals from other sources for financial gain.

The problem of referral for profit in health care delivery is addressed by

It is inaccurate, if not inappropriate, to refer to the business of health care as an industry. Those in the profession are strongly encouraged to focus on the special nature and status of health care and to challenge the use of the phrase, the health care industry, whenever it is used.

federal and state laws and by health professional codes of ethics. At the federal level, *Stark I and II*[1] are provisions within federal statutes that prohibit physician self-referral of Medicare- and Medicaid-funded patients for the following professional services, among others, in which the physician has a financial stake:

- Clinical laboratory services
- Durable medical equipment suppliers
- Occupational therapy
- Orthotics
- Physical therapy
- Prosthetics

Representative health professional codes of ethics also address business relations involving health professionals covered under their provisions. For example, the following sections of the *Guide for Professional Conduct* of the American Physical Therapy Association are illustrative.

Section 3.3A (Provision of Services): Physical therapists shall recognize the individual's freedom of choice in selection of physical therapy services.

Section 3.5 (Practice Arrangements):
A. Participation in a business, partnership, corporation, or other entity does not exempt the physical therapist, whether employer, partner, or stockholder, either individually or collectively, from the obligation of promoting and maintaining the ethical principles of the Association.
B. Physical therapists shall advise their employer(s) of any employer practice that causes a physical therapist to be in conflict with the ethical principles of the Association. *Physical therapist employees shall* attempt to *rectify aspects of their employment that are in conflict with the ethical principles of the Association* [emphasis added].

Section 5.2 (Business Practices/Fee Arrangements):
A. Physical therapists shall not:
1. Directly or indirectly request, receive, or participate in the dividing, transferring, assigning, or rebating of an unearned fee.
2. Profit by means of a credit or other valuable consideration, such as an unearned commission, discount, or gratuity in connection with furnishing physical therapy services.
B. Unless laws impose restrictions to the contrary, physical therapists who provide physical therapy services in a business entity may pool fees and moneys received. Physical therapists may divide or apportion these fees and moneys in accordance with the business agreement.
C. Physical therapists may enter into agreements with organizations to provide physical therapy services if such agreements do not violate the ethical principles of the Association.

Section 5.4 (Gifts and Other Considerations)
A. Physical therapists shall not accept nor offer gifts or other considerations with obligatory conditions attached.
B. Physical therapists shall not accept nor offer gifts or other considerations that affect *or give an objective appearance of affecting* their professional judgment [emphasis added].

Section 7.1B (Consumer Protection): Physical therapists may not participate in *any* arrangements in which patients are exploited due to the referring sources enhancing their personal incomes as a result of referring, prescribing, or recommending physical therapy.

Section 7.2 (Disclosure): The physical therapist shall disclose to the patient if the referring practitioner derives any compensation from the provision of physical therapy. The physical therapist shall *ensure* that the individual has a freedom of choice in selecting a provider of physical therapy [emphasis added].

Note that the *Guide for Professional Conduct* of the American Physical Therapy Association twice addresses the concern for patient freedom of choice in selecting providers of physical therapy services (sections 3.3A and 7.2). In fact, section 7.2 of the *Guide for Professional Conduct* imposes an affirmative obligation on clinical and managerial physical therapists to ensure patient freedom of choice in selecting a physical therapist.

Section 3.5 (Exploitation of Patients) of the *Guide for Conduct of the Affiliate Member* also establishes a professional ethical standard for physical therapist assistants regarding patient protection from exploitation. It reads:

Physical therapist assistants shall not participate in *any* arrangements in which patients are exploited. Such arrangements include (among others) situations in which referring sources enhance their personal incomes as a result of referring, delegating, prescribing, or recommending physical therapy [emphasis added].

This provision creates independent professional duties on the part of physical therapist assistants to protect patients from exploitation by anyone—including supervising physical therapists—and not to comply with illegal or unethical treatment orders that exploit patients under their care.

Similarly, Principles 1B and 5B of the *Occupational Therapy Code of Ethics* provide guidance for occupational therapy personnel, prohibiting patient financial exploitation and mandating disclosure of conflicts of interest between providers and patients, respectively.

Selected provisions of the *Canons of Ethical Conduct* of the American Board for Certification in Orthotics and Prosthetics also provide guidance regarding professional practice arrangements and affiliations. Canon 3.5 (Fees and Compensation) reads in pertinent part:

> The orthotist and prosthetist shall never place his or her own financial interest above the welfare of the patient.

This language, reiterating the fiduciary duty owed by orthotists and prosthetists to their patients, is one of the most powerful **directive** professional ethical provisions in any health professional code of ethics.

Similarly, the *Canons of Ethical Conduct* delineates in Canon 3.6 the prohibition against participating in patient referral for profit and imposes the affirmative professional ethical obligations on orthotists and prosthetists to "refer all patients to the most cost beneficial service provider" and to "disclose to [patients, when applicable] that the referring practitioner derives income from the provision of [orthotic or prosthetic] services."

Contractual Issues

Contracting issues impact all health professional relationships. In a contract, two or more parties possessing legal capacity to contract voluntarily enter into a binding legal agreement, supported by mutual consideration. Contracts may be express (i.e., explicit) or implied from the conduct of the parties and related circumstances. To be enforceable under law, contracts must not involve illegal matters and must not be found to be violative of public policy. For more detailed information on contract law, see *Promoting Legal Awareness in Physical and Occupational Therapy* (Scott R, St Louis, 1997, Mosby, chapter 5).

Although the law and health professional codes of ethics are especially protective of patient rights incident to health care services contracts, these sources of obligation provide less protection for business professionals contracting with one another for services, as in contracts for employment. In these latter areas, the law and ethics codes largely allow professional parties to bargain freely, within the constraints of legality and acceptable public policy, and to enjoy the fruits (or bear the consequences) of their agreements.

Although it may not always be the most socially responsible course of action, it is neither a violation of law or professional or business ethics for parties to attempt to secure the best possible bargain for themselves in their business contracts. In fact, Americans expect business contractual parties to maximize their position under contract, hence the current popular phrase, "Show me the money."[2]

Health professional employers and employees and related business people share the legal and ethical obligations not to exact contractual promises from one

Two or more health professionals possessing legal capacity to contract voluntarily may enter into an express or implied legal agreement, supported by mutual consideration.

another by coercion, deceit, duress, extortion, or undue influence, or to take advantage of parties' known incapacities. Beyond these considerations, however, professional parties to health services contracts bear personal legal and ethical responsibility to protect their own interests. All parties to health professional services contracts should, at a minimum, perform the following:

- Engage in real bargaining with the other contractual party or parties
- Reduce all business contracts to writing
- Carefully review written contracts affecting them, and reject by striking out provisions unacceptable to them before signing
- Have personal (or institutional, as applicable) legal counsel review important contracts before signing

There is shared legal and ethical obligations not to exact contractual promises through coercion, deceit, duress, extortion, or undue influence, or to take advantage of parties' known incapacities. Beyond these considerations, however, professional parties bear legal and ethical responsibility to protect their own interests.

Consider the following illustrative case examples:

An employment contract between an occupational therapist and a managed care organization (drafted by the employer's attorney) clearly provides for a waiver on the part of the employer for vicarious (indirect) liability on the part of the employer for the occupational therapist–employee's conduct within the scope of employment. The occupational therapist signs the agreement and, in a subsequent malpractice lawsuit, learns that his professional liability insurance policy is void because he waived vicarious liability on the part of his employer.

Was the conduct of the employer unethical? No. Absent a violation of law, an express professional or business ethical standard, or a public policy, the employer and employee each have the right to maximize their relative positions under the contract. The occupational therapist in this case had the duty to carefully read the contract and have his attorney review it before signing.

A physical therapist signs an employment contract with a national professional corporation, which contains the following covenant not to compete: The employee agrees, upon termination of this employee-employer relationship, not to engage in the practice of physical therapy within the state for a period of 5 years.

Is inclusion of the non-compete clause in the contract by the employer unethical? No. The non-compete clause is ethical unless the employer is aware or was advised by counsel that such a provision is illegal. A covenant or contractual promise not to compete, although technically a restraint of trade (which would normally be prohibited under federal antitrust laws, as violative of public policy), is accepted as legitimate in most states as a reasonable means to protect an employer's legitimate business interests.[3] As stated in Chapter 5, a covenant not to compete in an employment contract typically must meet four criteria to be valid and enforceable:

- It must be supported by consideration, that is, the covenant not to compete must have been made as part of a bargained-for exchange, and value must have been given by the employer in exchange for the employee's promise not to compete.
- A covenant not to compete must be reasonable in three areas[4]:
  - ▲ Geographic area of practice restriction
  - ▲ Specific practice restrictions
  - ▲ Time

As in the previous example, the physical therapist had the affirmative duty as a party with full contractual capacity to carefully read the contract and have his legal advisor review it before signing. The employer had no legal or ethical duty, or place, to advise the therapist on the non-compete clause in the contract.

Professional Advertising

When it comes to advertising professional health care services, the traditional adage of *caveat emptor* ("Let the buyer beware") is tempered by legal and ethical considerations favoring patient rights. Until the late 1970s, health professional ethics codes, and those of the legal profession, proscribed professional advertising.

Advertising in any form by health care and legal professionals was formerly considered inappropriate for a number of reasons. It was argued that advertising health care and legal services had an adverse effect on professionalism; was misleading; and engendered undesirable economic consequences, including increased overhead cost passed on to consumers and the creation of a substantial entry barrier to junior professional colleagues attempting to enter or penetrate a market. In 1977, these arguments were systematically addressed and refuted by the United States Supreme Court in *Bates and Van O'Steen v. State Bar of Arizona,*[5] the landmark legal case involving professional advertising.

In *Bates,* the United States Supreme Court held that the advertising of professional services fell within the rubric of First Amendment free speech rights. Specifically, the Court declared that truthful advertising about the availability and cost

Health care professionals should ensure that their business contracts are: (1) in writing; (2) clearly reflect the intentions of the parties to the contract; and (3) carefully read by them and reviewed by their personal legal counsel before being signed.

of professional service delivery serves an important societal interest—to ensure that consumers make informed decisions about professional services based on readily available, complete, and reliable information.

Because professional advertising is a form of *commercial speech,* it does not enjoy the broadest constitutional protection otherwise afforded to political or literary speech under the First Amendment. Government entities are free to regulate professional advertising to prevent the dissemination of misleading, deceptive, or false advertising, and advertisements for illegal activities (i.e., regulated health services rendered by unauthorized providers). As with other forms of protected speech, states may impose reasonable restrictions on the time, place, and manner of professional advertising.

Forms of health care professional advertising that might be prohibited as misleading, deceptive, or false could include advertisements that compare the relative quality of services offered among competitors (*comparative competitor claims*). In addition to being subject to constitutionally permissible state regulation, such advertisements might expose the advertising professional to common-law business tort liability (discussed in this chapter).

Subsequent to *Bates,* many health disciplines revised their ethics codes to reflect the change in legal status of professional advertising. For example, Sections 6.2 B and C of the American Physical Therapy Association's *Guide for Professional Conduct* reads:

B. Physical therapists may advertise their services to the public.
C. Physical therapists shall not use, or participate in the use of, any form of communication containing a false, plagiarized, fraudulent, misleading, deceptive, unfair, or sensational statement or claim.

Principle 5C of the *Occupational Therapy Code of Ethics* does not address professional advertising directly but reads in pertinent part:

Occupational therapy personnel shall refrain from using or participating in the use of any form of communication that contains false, fraudulent, deceptive, or unfair statements or claims.

Canon 3.11 of the *Canons of Ethical Conduct* of the American Board for Certification in Orthotics and Prosthetics also provides guidance on the ethically permissible scope of professional advertising by orthotists and prosthetists. It reads in pertinent part:

Orthotists and prosthetists shall not use, nor participate in any use of, any form of communication containing a false, fraudulent, misleading, deceptive,

The advertising of professional services requires a balance between legal and ethical considerations and the right of professionals to free speech; such a balance is not always easy to maintain.

unfair or sensational statement or claim. Orthotists and prosthetists shall not provide any consideration to any member of the press, radio or television, or other communication medium in exchange for professional publicity in a news item. All advertisements shall be identified as advertisements unless it is absolutely clear from the context that it is a paid advertisement.

The advertising of professional services requires a balance between legal and ethical considerations and the right of professionals to free speech. Such a balance is not always easy to maintain.

Fraud, Waste, and Abuse

Health care delivery is perhaps the most regulated commercial business in the United States. Federal health programs, including Medicare, Medicaid, and TriCare (for military beneficiaries), are the responsibility of the Department of Health and Human Services (HHS). The Health Care Financing Administration (HCFA) is the agency within HHS directly responsible for administering these health care programs.

Medicare is the largest payer of health care services in the United States and reimburses health providers and institutions more than $150 billion annually, a figure that is increasing at 10.5 percent per year.[6] The Office of the Inspector General (OIG) of HHS bears primary responsibility for ensuring compliance by providers with statutory and administrative Medicare mandates. A finding of Medicare "program-related misconduct" (e.g., the filing of fraudulent claims for reimbursement[7]) can lead to mandatory exclusion from participation in federally funded health programs administratively and to criminal prosecution for fraud by the Criminal Division of the Department of Justice. Not only are providers subject to criminal prosecution for fraud, but contracting entities that process claims are also. In the first case of its kind, a Medicare claims administrator employed by Blue Shield of California agreed to plead guilty to three criminal counts of conspiracy and obstructing federal Medicare audits incident to the activities of six of its employees.[8]

In fiscal year 1996, HCFA overpaid health care providers approximately 23 billion dollars, according to a comprehensive Medicare audit.[9] As a result, the Office of the Inspector General of HHS has initiated widespread fraud investigations and inquiries,

Fraud: **The intentional false representation or concealment of a material fact, designed to deceive another person or entity, which causes that person or entity to act (or not act) in some manner, to the victim's legal detriment. Commission of fraud constitutes a violation of civil and criminal law, licensure and certification regulations, and professional and business ethics.**

127

pursuant to the False Claims Act, Stark Laws, and the Medicare and Medicaid Patient Protection Act (also known as the "Anti-Kickback Law"). In August 1997, the American Hospital Association, on behalf of over 5000 member hospitals, beseeched HHS for a 6-month moratorium on new fraud investigations so that hospitals could assess and improve compliance with federal statutes and HHS regulations.[10]

Impaired Providers

Health care providers impaired by drugs (including alcohol), mental distress, or other causes pose a serious risk of substantial harm to patients under their care and research subjects; to colleagues, visitors and others; and to themselves. For that reason, professional ethical standards and licensure and certification regulations and other state and federal laws make mandatory the reporting of suspected impairment by peers of the subject.

Policy statements of representative rehabilitation professions[11,12] make clear that health care professionals have the personal ethical responsibility to recognize the signs and symptoms of possible abuse affecting themselves and to refrain from carrying out interventions that might harm patients or others. Section 3.1D of the *Guide for Professional Conduct* of the American Physical Therapy Association formally enunciates this standard as follows:

> The physical therapist shall not provide physical therapy services to a patient while under the influence of a substance that impairs his or her ability to do so safely.

Because a primary purpose of health professional codes of ethics is patient and public protection, it is expected that ethics codes will require peer reporting of unethical, illegal conduct, or suspected incompetence. All four representative ethics codes (*Canons of Ethical Conduct* of the American Board for Certification in Orthotics and Prosthetics [Canon 6.1], *Guide for Professional Conduct* [Section 7.1] and *Guide for Conduct of the Affiliate Member* [Section 6.1] of the American Physical Therapy Association, and *Occupational Therapy Code of Ethics* [Principle 6C]) so provide.

Canon 6.1 of the *Canons of Ethical Conduct* of the American Board for Certification in Orthotics and Prosthetics interposes an important, nondirective prereporting step, imploring orthotists and prosthetists first, whenever feasible, to direct their concerns about a peer's or professional colleague's patient care activities to the source of the problem. It reads in pertinent part:

> Concerns regarding patient care provided by other professionals should be addressed directly to that professional rather than to the patient.

Summary

Health care services delivery, though a professional business pursuit, is not an everyday *industry*. Because of the unique responsibilities of health care professionals, special status and ethical and legal duties are imposed upon them. Health professional practice, however, must be approached from a business perspective to survive and thrive in the current managed care environment.

Legal and professional ethical standards prohibit the referral of patients for profit (including self-referral to entities in which the referral source has a financial stake) and restrict the offering and accepting of gifts incident to practice. Health care professionals have self-policing ethical duties, including responsibility for knowing the provisions in their business contracts before signing them and recognizing signs and symptoms of impairment that might affect professional judgment and patient safety and the safety of others.

Ethical standards require health care providers to report suspected impairment in professional colleagues to appropriate authorities. Although this reporting duty must be taken seriously, concerns should be first addressed, whenever possible, to the source of the concern as a matter of professional respect and courtesy.

Cases and Questions

1. A physical therapist in private practice in a medium-sized town habitually pays to have lunch delivered on a weekly basis to potential physician referral sources and to the staff in those physicians' offices as a matter of "business goodwill." Over the course of three months, the therapist has lunches delivered to the offices of all twelve physicians in town, after which the therapist begins the process anew. The therapist also routinely pays for dinners and/or drinks for referring physicians and their guests any time the therapist sees one of them in local restaurants. What, if anything, is wrong with this marketing practice?

2. Patient "no-shows" for appointments is a problem affecting all health care disciplines. D, a physical therapist–employee of XYZ Company, a physical therapist–owned private practice, is directed by M, the owner of XYZ, to bill third-party payers at minimal rates for no-show patients to minimize financial losses associated with loss of revenue associated with these patients. Is this acceptable?

Suggested Answers for Cases and Questions

1. Although marketing of services inherently involves solicitation of business, these marketing practices may be violative of Section 5.4 of the *Guide for Professional Conduct* of the American Physical Therapy Association, which reads:

continued

Suggested Answers for Cases and Questions—cont'd

Section 5.4 (Gifts and Other Considerations)
  A. Physical therapists shall not accept nor offer gifts or other considerations with obligatory conditions attached.
  B. Physical therapists shall not accept nor offer gifts or other considerations that affect or give an objective appearance of affecting their professional judgment.
  The physical therapist should seek an advisory ethics opinion from the Judicial Committee of the American Physical Therapy Association before proceeding further.

2. Billing for patient care for no-shows constitutes reimbursement fraud, a violation of law and professional ethics.

References

1. 42 United States Code Section 1395nn.

2. Dialogue from the film *Jerry Maguire*, 1996, TriStar Films.

3. Wallen E: A restrictive covenant can lessen practice's risk of losing patients, *Physicians Financial News* 26, May 1991.

4. Freed C, Martinez WL: Non-compete covenant has to be reasonable, *San Antonio Medical Gazette* 8, Jun 9-15, 1993

5. *Bates and Van O'Steen v. State Bar of Arizona*, 433 U.S. 350 (1977).

6. Anders G, McGinley L: Managed eldercare: HMOs are signing up new class of member: the group in Medicare, *Wall Street Journal* A1, A5, Apr 27, 1995.

7. Scott RW: *Legal aspects of documenting patient care*, Gaithersburg, Md, 1994, Aspen Publishers, p 201.

8. Rundle RL: Medicare fraud case draws guilty plea, *Wall Street Journal* B2, Apr 29, 1996.

9. Anders G: Improper Medicare spending is frequent, *Wall Street Journal* A2, Jun 11, 1997.

10. Hospitals seek moratorium on investigations of fraud, *PT Bulletin* 10, Aug 1, 1997.

11. American Occupational Therapy Association: *Guidelines to the occupational therapy code of ethics: draft II*, Bethesda, Md, 1997, AOTA, p 9.

12. Association of Rehabilitation Nurses: *Position statement on the impaired nurse*, Glenview, Ill, 1984, The Association.

Suggested Readings

Anders G: Story of Jack Mills is lesson in the difficulty of policing Medicare, *Wall Street Journal* A1, A6, Jul 21, 1997.

Bates and Van O'Steen v. State Bar of Arizona, 433 U.S. 350 (1977).

Eisler P: Studies: home care groups guilty of billions in Medicare fraud, *USA Today* 4A, Jul 28, 1997.

Furrow BR, Johnson SH, Jost TS, Schwartz RL: *Health law: cases, materials and problems*, ed 2, St Paul, Minn, 1991, West Publishing, p 55-57.

American Occupational Therapy Association: *Guidelines to the occupational therapy code of ethics: draft II,* Bethesda, Md, 1997, AOTA.

Kurlander SS: Fraud and abuse issues, *Rehab Economics* 5(3):105, 1997.

Lewis K: Physical therapy contracts, *Clinical Management* 12(6):14, 1992.

Medicare fraud still pervasive despite efforts, *PT Bulletin* 12, Jun 6, 1997.

Murer CG: Medicare fraud and abuse, *Rehab Management* 103-104, Jun/Jul, 1997.

Association of Rehabilitation Nurses: *Position statement on the impaired nurse,* Glenview, Ill, 1984, The Association.

Rohland P: Physical therapists under close observation: knowledge best tool in avoiding workers' comp fraud, *Advance for Physical Therapists* 8:23. Mar 10, 1997.

Schmeltzer, Aptaker, Shepard: *Civil money penalties reporter: Medicare/Medicaid fraud & abuse* 1-4, (Spring)1997.

Scott RW: *Legal aspects of documenting patient care,* Gaithersburg, Md, 1994, Aspen Publishers.

Scott RW: *Promoting legal awareness in physical and occupational therapy,* St Louis, 1997, Mosby.

Skoler DL: Health care fraud & abuse, *Public Lawyer* 5(1):5, 1997.

Sexual Harassment and Misconduct

7

This chapter addresses the mixed legal-professional ethical issues of sexual harassment and sexual misconduct. The chapter commences by describing how provider-patient sexual activity denigrates from the customary professional relationship and from the provider's fiduciary duties owed to the patient. The section also demonstrates how such activity violates the four foundational biomedical ethical principles. Sexual misconduct in general is explored next, focusing on sexual assault and battery and putative *consensual* meretricious relationships between health care professionals and patients. Discussion of workplace sexual harassment follows, including the Equal Employment Opportunity Commission's definition of sexual harassment and a detailed examination of *quid pro quo* and hostile work environment sexual harassment. The chapter concludes with a discussion of special duties and problems involving health care academicians, clinical faculty, and health professional students.

Nature of the Problem

Sexual harassment and misconduct in the health care delivery environment are problems that are, or should be, a grave concern to health care educators, administrators, clinical managers and professionals, professional students, patients, and relevant others. Allegations made by patients of sexual misconduct on the part of clinical health care professionals constitute one of the fastest growing bases for health care malpractice claims.[1]

In only a few business relationships—including health care delivery—are professionals privileged to enter into clients' personal and intimate zones.[2] When a health care provider breaches the legal and professional ethical duties owed to a patient and commits sexual battery or engages in sexual harassment of a patient, it reflects extremely negatively, not only on the perpetrator personally, but also on the perpetrator's health care discipline and even on health care professions generally. Sexual harassment and misconduct committed by providers against patients evince the greatest degree of disrespect for the foundational biomedical ethical principles that undergird professional ethical responsibilities in patient care delivery.

Commission of sexually related misconduct shows complete disregard for patient autonomy or self-determination. Patients commonly display **transference** emotions directed toward their health care providers. Sometimes, these transference emotions are manifested as romantic feelings. Providers, as fiduciaries toward their patients, are not privileged to engage in reciprocal **countertransference,** since they are bound to refrain from such conduct by professional ethical and legal standards, their professional educational instruction, and customary practice.

When health care providers engage in sexual misconduct with patients, they violate the duty to "do no (intentional) harm" to patients under their care (**nonmaleficence**). It is always adverse to a patient's best interests (**beneficence**) when the patient's health care provider allows a professional relationship to denigrate into a personal and intimate one. Finally, it is simply unfair (**justice**) that a health care professional would breach the special trust embodied in him or her as a fiduciary and become enamored of a patient under his or her care.

Sexual Misconduct Involving Health Care Professionals and Patients

Whereas all sexual harassment entails sexual misconduct, not all sexually related misconduct involves sexual harassment. Sexual harassment normally involves conduct of a sexual nature that affects the productivity, work product, morale, or physical and/or mental well-being of a worker in an employment setting. (Sexual harassment is discussed in greater detail in this chapter.) Sexual misconduct, on the other hand, is defined broadly enough to encompass all illicit and unethical sexually ori-

When a health care provider commits sexual battery or engages in sexual harassment of a patient, it reflects extremely negatively, not only on the perpetrator personally, but also on the perpetrator's health care discipline and even on health care professions generally.

ented behavior in any given setting. In the health care environment, sexual misconduct allegations may arise from relations involving professionals, students, patients and their significant others, and anyone else present in such settings. Sexual misconduct allegations may involve relations that are consensual, as well as nonconsensual, in nature.

Rehabilitation professionals are sometimes referred to as *hands-on* health care providers. These professionals experience among the closest and most intense professional relationships with their patients of any profession—in large part because of the extensive amount of time devoted to their patients during the process of rehabilitation. Also, rehabilitation professionals and their assistants and other support personnel often become privy to a great deal of personal information about their patients, which is relayed to them during evaluation, treatment, or in other professional-patient dialogue.

From a legal point of view, there are two broad classifications of sexual misconduct involving health professionals and patients. The first type is nonconsensual **sexual assault** or **battery,** which may be defined as:

> Any nonconsensual, intentional touching of a patient's or a health care provider's sexual or other body parts (or clothing), with the intent to arouse or gratify the sexual desires of either party to the relationship, or for the express purpose of patient sexual abuse.[3]

Commission by a health care provider of nonconsensual sexual battery upon a patient can give rise to civil liability for intentional conduct-based health care malpractice; criminal liability; adverse administrative and organizational action affecting licensure and/or certification, institutional credentials, and employment; and adverse action before professional associations for violations of professional ethics. A finding of civil liability against a health care professional may be followed by an award of **punitive,** or punishment-focused, money damages in favor of the victim, as well as the customary compensatory damages for associated medical expenses, lost earnings, and pain and suffering. In such a case, the health care professional may be personally liable for the civil judgment, because in many cases, professional liability insurance does not indemnify an insured for malicious misconduct or punitive damages.

The other type of health care-setting sexual misconduct involves putative "consensual" intimate relations between health care providers and patients. In such a relationship, a patient becomes infatuated with, or enamored of, his or her health care provider, with follow-on reciprocal display of emotions by the provider who is the object of the patient's affections. Because of transference emotions, the inherent vulnerability of patients, which are dependent upon health care providers for care and support, and the fiduciary duties of trust and good faith, which are incumbent upon providers, the concept of consent on the part of patients to meretricious sex-

A finding of civil liability against a health care professional may be followed by an award of punitive damages in favor of the victim, as well as the customary compensatory damages for associated medical expenses, lost earnings, and pain and suffering.

ual relations with health care professionals responsible for their care has no real meaning. Health care professionals alone bear full legal and professional ethical responsibility for the creation and maintenance of such relationships. Patients are not bound to defined standards of conduct under professional codes of ethics, as are health care professionals.

Section 1.3 (Patient Relations) of the *Guide for Professional Conduct* of the American Physical Therapy Association establishes the standard for physical therapist–patient relationships, as follows:

> Physical therapists *shall not* [emphasis added] engage in any sexual relationship or activity, whether consensual or nonconsensual, with any patient while a physical therapist–patient relationship exists.

Principle 1B of the American Occupational Therapy Association's *Occupational Therapy Code of Ethics* creates a similar standard for occupational therapy practitioners. It reads, in pertinent part:

> Occupational therapy personnel shall maintain relationships that do not exploit the recipient of services *sexually* [emphasis added]...or in any other manner.

Not addressed in the above professional ethical standards is guidance concerning suggested waiting periods after severance of health professional–patient relationships, before commencing intimate relationships. Some authorities suggest a minimum 6-month waiting period.[4]

Prudent clinical risk management is designed to meet providers' legal and professional ethical duties to patients and to minimize or avoid liability exposure and ethical complaints. Simple risk management measures that can decrease the incidence of sexual misconduct allegations by patients include, among others:

- Providing, upon patient request, a same-gender chaperone during patient evaluation and treatment or in response to the reasonable request of an evaluating or treating health care provider
- Implementing procedures such as a "knock-and-enter" policy, under which staff may enter a closed door during patient evaluation or treatment after due notice
- Establishing detailed patient informed consent policies concerning intensive, hands-on evaluative and treatment procedures, so that patients possess maximum information and so that misunderstandings about the nature of therapeutic touch are minimized

All sexual conduct with patients should be considered nonconsensual.

- Providing ongoing continuing education for staff, contract professionals, consultants, and relevant others, concerning sexual harassment and misconduct, and facility policies in these areas.

Workplace Sexual Harassment

Though sexual harassment has long been a widespread problem affecting productivity, morale, and every other aspect of interpersonal relations in the workplace, only recently have allegations of sexual harassment lodged against prominent public officials brought this problem "out of the closet" and into every boardroom, work setting, and living room in the United States and elsewhere.

The Equal Employment Opportunity Commission (EEOC), the federal regulatory agency responsible for promulgating national policy concerning workplace sexual harassment and enforcing its provisions, administratively or in court, defines[5] sexual harassment as:

> Unwelcome sexual advances, requests for sexual favors, and other verbal or physical conduct of a sexual nature, when (1) submission to such conduct is made either explicitly or implicitly a term or condition of employment; (2) submission to or rejection of such conduct by an individual is used as a basis for employment decisions affecting such individual; or (3) such conduct has the purpose or effect of unreasonably interfering with an individual's work performance or creating an intimidating, hostile, or offensive work environment.

The EEOC definition of sexual harassment has a dual focus on (1) the types of inappropriate conduct that constitutes sexual harassment and (2) the possible adverse employment consequences for victims of sexual harassment and for others in the workplace. Conduct that constitutes sexual harassment could include:

- Unwelcome comments of a sexual nature about a victim's person or body parts
- Solicitation of others for sexual relations
- Inappropriate touching of another person on a private area of his or her body with the intent to arouse or gratify sexual desires (i.e., commission of sexual battery)

Employment consequences fall into two categories, adverse employment decisions resulting from *quid pro quo* situations and hostile work environments. *Quid pro quo* describes a situation in which a victim's response to sexual harassment is the basis for employment-related decisions involving the victim or other workers. A *quid pro quo* complaint typically is lodged either by an employee who has been denied opportunities because he or she refused a perpetrator's sexual advances or by an employee who has been denied opportunities because another employee obtained those opportunities by submitting to a perpetrator's sexual advances. An example of a *quid pro quo* sexual harassment situation would be the case in which an employer's decision to fund a staff occupational therapist's attendance at a professional conference depended on whether the occupational therapist submitted to the employer's sexual advances.

In a hostile work environment scenario, sexual harassment unreasonably interferes with either the victim's or another person's work performance. Complaints related to hostile work environments can be made by any person in the workplace who is reasonably offended by a perpetrator's sexual harassment (of the complainant or of another person in the work setting) and whose work is impeded by that harassment. An example of a hostile work environment sexual harassment situation would be the case in which a certified rehabilitation aide is unable to concentrate on patient care activities because of the misconduct of a licensed rehabilitation supervisory professional who is making sexual advances toward a patient.

The EEOC and the courts adjudicating sexual harassment cases traditionally have utilized the "ordinary reasonable person" standard to assess whether an individual's conduct constitutes sexual harassment. This is the same standard commonly used to determine whether a defendant in a civil tort (e.g., health care malpractice) case violated a duty owed to a plaintiff. Under this standard, as applied in a sexual harassment case, a trier of fact (judge or jury) places himself or herself into the shoes of an ethereal "person of ordinary care and diligence"[6] and determines how such a person would be likely to perceive the conduct in issue and decides the case accordingly.

The problem with the traditional "ordinary reasonable person" standard is that it frequently is translated into a "reasonable man" standard, with the result that the trier of fact assesses interpersonal conduct exclusively from a man's point of view. To ensure that a gender-neutral standard is applied in administrative and legal sexual harassment cases, some federal courts have established a modified standard that eventually may supplant the traditional standard of review. Under this modified standard, the trier of fact still places himself or herself into the shoes of an "ordinary reasonable person" when determining whether specific conduct constitutes sexual harassment, but the "ordinary reasonable person" must be of the same gender as the alleged victim of sexual harassment or misconduct.

Expert testimony has been presented in sexual harassment cases to support the notion that men and women view sexually oriented conduct—in the workplace and elsewhere—differently. Testifying in *Robinson v. Jacksonville Shipyards,*[7] Alison Wetherfield of the National Organization for Women's Legal Defense and Education Fund cited a study in which 75 percent of men polled said that they were flattered by sexual advances by women in the workplace; only 15 percent claimed that

> Complaints related to hostile work environments can be made by any person in the workplace who is reasonably offended by a perpetrator's sexual harassment (of the complainant or of another person in the work setting) and whose work is impeded by that harassment.

they would be offended by such conduct. Of women surveyed, however, 75 percent stated that they would be offended by sexually oriented conduct in the workplace.[8] In *Robinson,* the court employed an "ordinary reasonable woman" standard to hold an employer responsible for the sexually harassing conduct of male employees toward a female co-worker.

Supporting Alison Wetherfield's assertion that men and women view sexually oriented conduct differently is a recently reported study done by the spousal research team of Struckman-Johnson and Struckman-Johnson, reported in 1994 in the journal, *Sex Roles.*[9] In a study of 277 college men, subjects were asked to imagine that they were the target of unsolicited sexual advances from casual female acquaintances. Conduct to be imagined ranged from a gentle touch on the genitals, to a push, to coercion with and without a deadly weapon. Nearly 25 percent of the men stated that they would willingly continue sexual activity with an "attractive" female aggressor, even if coerced by the assailant with a deadly weapon.

In another legal case, *Ellison v. Brady,*[10] a federal appeals court evaluated what were described as "bizarre," repetitive, unwelcome love letters written by a male co-worker to a woman in a federal government office. The lower court found that the man's conduct did not constitute sexual harassment. In reversing that decision, the appellate court adopted an "ordinary reasonable woman" standard to assess whether the letters constituted sexual harassment.

An excellent model for assessing interpersonal conduct is the one developed by the United States Navy[11] after the Tailhook convention in which a number of male officers were accused of sexually harassing female colleagues at an aviator's convention at the Las Vegas Hilton Hotel. This model categorizes conduct as either:

- "Green light," that is, interpersonal conduct that is clearly acceptable behavior in the eyes of an "ordinary reasonable person" of either gender
- "Yellow light," that is, conduct that may be unacceptable in the eyes of some "reasonable" persons of the same gender as the target of the conduct
- "Red light," that is, conduct that is always unacceptable in the eyes of an "ordinary reasonable person" of the same gender as the target of the conduct

"Green light" conduct might include such things as complimenting a colleague about his or her dress in an inoffensive and nondiscriminatory manner. "Yellow light" behavior might include soliciting a date with a co-worker for the first time. "Red light" behavior includes such conduct as repeated solicitations for a date after rejection, indecent exposure, and sexual assault or battery. Media depictions of workplace sexual assault and battery, such as presented in the film, "Disclosure,"[12] promote the trivialization of serious sexual misconduct in the public's eye by labeling it merely as "sexual harassment." Such serious, felonious sexual misconduct involves conduct more egregious than simple "sexual harassment."

In the workplace, managers bear the formidable responsibility of ferreting out, eliminating, and preventing sexual harassment. The buck *does* stop at the manager's desk. Managers may even be held liable for sexual harassment of which they are unaware, especially if the organization or work unit does not have in place a reporting or grievance mechanism for receiving and investigating complaints of sexual harassment. Management also is liable when it fails to take appropriate action on a complaint found to be valid at the conclusion of an investigation.[13] Managers are not free to assume an "ostrich defense." They will be held responsible for what they should have observed and corrected.[14] Specific management responsibilities regarding sexual harassment include:

- *Sensitizing and educating employees about what constitutes sexual harassment; how men and women may differ in their attitudes toward sexual conduct; and the types of conduct that reasonable persons might find offensive.* This process not only should be a part of new employee orientations, it also should be regularly reinforced as continuing for all employees. Managers might wish to consult with human resource management specialists to lead sessions at which employees are given information about current administrative and legal sexual harassment cases and are asked to participate in group cooperative learning processes, such as brainstorming about what interpersonal conduct constitutes permissible and impermissible behavior in the workplace.[15]

- *Expressing strong disapproval of sexual harassment and developing and enforcing appropriate sanctions to stop sexual harassment whenever it is found to exist.* Managers are responsible for taking immediate action to stop known sexual harassment, regardless of who the perpetrator[16] or the victim might be. Reporting, investigation, and grievance procedures for internal resolution of sexual harassment complaints should be in place. Managers must be fair and impartial in their investigations of such complaints, respecting the rights of all parties involved, to the maximum extent possible.[17] If employees and others view management's commitment as strong, the investigatory process as equitable, and the awarding of sanctions as appropriate, then minor complaints stand a better chance of being resolved at the organizational level instead of through the EEOC or the courts.

In the workplace, managers bear the responsibility of ferreting out, eliminating, and preventing sexual harassment—the buck stops at the manager's desk.

• *Alerting employees, as required by federal law, of their right to initiate formal charges with the EEOC.* Although victims of sexual harassment should be encouraged to resolve grievances at the lowest appropriate level, under the EEOC sex-discrimination guidelines, managers are responsible for making their employees aware of their right to pursue unresolved complaints at higher administrative or legal levels. Making employees aware of their rights could be done as part of the sensitization and ongoing educational processes. In addition, managers should ensure that both a statement of employees' rights and the organization's policy statement on sexual harassment, with a clear description of the internal grievance process, is posted in a prominent place.

Do Title VII of the Civil Rights Act of 1964, the EEOC's Sex Discrimination Guidelines, and professional ethics standards afford protection to victims of same-gender sexual harassment? Currently, it is uncertain whether federal civil rights laws provide protection to victims of same-gender workplace sexual harassment; however, health professional ethics standards clearly do offer such protection.

For example, Section 1.1C of the *Guide for Professional Conduct* of the American Physical Therapy Association requires physical therapists not to "engage in conduct that constitutes harassment or abuse of, or discrimination against, colleagues...." This ethical provision does not exclude any class of victim of potential abuse, discrimination, or harassment from its scope of coverage. (Section 2.1C of the *Guide for Conduct of the Affiliate Member* establishes an identical professional ethical standard for physical therapist assistants.)

Similarly, Canon 1.2 of the *Canons of Ethical Conduct* of the American Board for Certification in Orthotics and Prosthetics requires orthotists and prosthetists to conform their professional conduct to the "customs and practices of the profession," and to the requirements of law, including federal and state civil rights laws proscribing sexual harassment. (Principle 4A of the American Occupational Therapy Association's *Occupational Therapy Code of Ethics* creates a similar professional ethical standard for occupational therapy personnel.) Although the status of federal legal protections against same-gender sexual harassment may be in limbo, the customary practice of rehabilitation health professions no more permits same-gender sexual harassment than it does sexual harassment of colleagues of the opposite gender.

In June 1997, the United States Supreme Court agreed to decide whether Title VII of The Civil Rights Act of 1964 protects victims of sexual harassment who are of the same gender as the perpetrator of sexually oriented misconduct.[18] In *Oncale v. Sundowner Offshore Services, Inc.*,[19] a male employee sued his employer and

Although the status of federal legal protections against same-gender sexual harassment may be in limbo, the customary practice of rehabilitation health professions no more permits same-gender sexual harassment than it does sexual harassment of colleagues of the opposite gender.

male co-workers for alleged lewd and lascivious conduct and threats of homosexual rape while on the job on an offshore oil rig. The United States Court of Appeals, Fifth Circuit, ruled that same-gender sexual harassment is not protected under Title VII. (The Eighth Circuit, in *Quick v. Donaldson Company, Inc.,*[20] suggested that such misconduct is prohibited by Title VII.). The United States Supreme Court decision in *Oncale* in 1998 will hopefully resolve this controversy.

Special Issues in Health Professional Education Settings

Sexual harassment and misconduct issues in health professional educational settings primarily involve student-professor, student–clinical instructor, student-student, and student-patient scenarios. Because the representative professional codes of ethics are relatively ambiguous in their treatment of these issues, guidance on appropriate conduct derives largely from federal and state laws and customary practice patterns.

Health professional students are protected from sexual harassment and misconduct in educational settings not only by the Civil Rights Act of 1964 but also by Title IX of the Education Amendments of 1972.[21] Health professional academic and clinical educators should maintain the same formality in relationships with professional students as they maintain with patients to avoid misunderstandings and the appearance of impropriety.

Students must also be cognizant of their ethical duties to maintain appropriate relationships with faculty and patients. Although a majority of health professionals may have experienced inappropriate behaviors of a sexual nature on the part of patients under their care,[22] students (similar to clinical professionals) may also be the perpetrators of sexual misconduct upon patients. Consider the reported federal health care malpractice legal case, *Oslund v. United States.*[23] In this case, a patient sued the United States for the alleged sexual misconduct of an occupational therapy intern at a Veterans Administration hospital. The alleged misconduct involved a meretricious relationship between the student intern and the psychiatric patient, during which time one transferred genital herpes to the other. The federal district court ruled, in part, that the intern's otherwise confidential medical records were to be opened for the patient's attorney to determine when she developed and first sought treatment for herpes.

Clinical managers and instructors must be sure to include health professional students in the scope of coverage of their policy manuals prohibiting sexual contact between staff and patients, and orient students as to their responsibilities immediately upon arrival at the clinical sites. It is also prudent to have in place work rules prohibiting dating between staff and patients, as well as staff and students in the clinic.

Clinical managers and instructors must be sure to include health professional students in the scope of coverage of their policy manuals prohibiting sexual contact between staff and patients, and orient students as to their responsibilities immediately upon arrival at the clinical sites.

Summary

Sexual misconduct is inclusive of all forms of sexual harassment, but not the other way around. Both forms of misconduct evidence disrespect for victims, and both are disparaging, not only of perpetrators in the health care environment but of the perpetrators' disciplines and health care in general. Sexual exploitation of patients, colleagues, students, and others, is proscribed by law, customary practice, and professional ethical standards promulgated by professional associations of respective health care disciplines.

There are two types of sexual misconduct involving health care providers and patients: nonconsensual and putative consensual sex. Since patients display transference emotions toward their caregivers, the concept of consent to sexual relations has no real meaning. All sexual conduct with patients is therefore nonconsensual.

There are also two types of workplace sexual harassment: *quid pro quo*, or favorable employment considerations in exchange for sex, involving superiors and subordinates; and sexual harassment by a perpetrator of any person in the workplace, creating a hostile work environment and reasonably adversely affecting the work of a victim. The EEOC and federal courts have established legal standards regarding sexual harassment, which complement professional ethical standards promulgated by health professional associations across many disciplines.

Anyone can be a victim of sexual harassment, and everyone can be a perpetrator. Therefore every health care professional must be vigilant, but open, in professional relations with patients, colleagues, students, and others in the course of official duty.

Cases and Questions

1. P is a 36-year-old female physical therapist–MBA, who is employed as a regional facilities manager for XYZ Company, a national rehabilitation services corporation. D, an important business client of XYZ Company, makes an inappropriate pass at P during a business lunch and subsequently fondles her breasts in the parking lot after lunch. What action(s) should P take?

2. X, a male medical student affiliated with ABC Hospital, solicits a date from Y, a female occupational therapy intern working at the facility. Is X's conduct, per se, improper? Is it appropriate for X and Y to date?

Suggested Answers for Cases and Questions

1. The level of resolution of this problem depends a great deal on the kind of business organization that XYZ is. If XYZ Company fairly investigates P's complaint, takes no retaliatory action against her for filing a complaint, and

continued

takes appropriate action to P's reasonable satisfaction in resolving the problem, the issue may never rise to the level of an EEOC complaint. However, if P is coerced or attempted to be coerced into dropping her complaint, XYZ not only is breaching business and professional ethics, but it is also courting deservedly severe administrative or judicial sanctions for being a principal to D's sexual harassment. For an interesting analysis of a similar case and commentary from five business experts, see Magretta's "Will She Fit In?" (*Harvard Business Review* 75(2):18, 1997.)

2. Based on these facts alone, X's solicitation of a date with Y and the process of dating between X and Y are not improper. ABC Hospital and the students' respective schools may not be legally empowered to impose and enforce a dating ban between students (although they would be so empowered to disallow dating patients and probably dating between students and staff).

References

1. Susko K: Insurance and Member Benefits Service, *Personal communication,* Alexandria, Va, 1997, American Physical Therapy Association.

2. Purtilo R: *Health professional and patient interaction,* ed 4, Philadelphia, 1990, WB Saunders, p 149. The four physical zones of social interaction are: (1) the public zone, in which physical contact is unlikely; (2) the social zone, in which everyday office or school-setting interaction occurs; (3) the personal zone, in which face-to-face business transactions occur; and (4) the intimate zone, involving hands-on contact between two or more people, such as patient and health care provider(s).

3. See Model Penal Code, Section 213.4, American Law Institute, 1962.

4. Stromber CD, Haggarty DJ, Leibenluft RF, et al: Physical contact and sexual relations with patients. In *The psychologist's legal handbook,* Washington, DC, 1988, Council for National Register of Health Service Providers in Psychology, p 463. Of the total number of reported cases of sexual abuse involving psychiatrists and patients, 80 percent are estimated to involve male therapists and female patients; 13 percent, female therapists and female patients; 5 percent, male therapists and male patients; and 2 percent, female therapists and male patients. (Scott RW: Sexual misconduct, *PT Magazine of Physical Therapy* 1(1):78, 1993.)

5. Equal Employment Opportunity Commission: *Sex discrimination guidelines,* EEOC 29 Code of Federal Regulations 1604.11, Federal Register, 45:74677, 1980.

6. *Black's law dictionary,* ed 3, St Paul, Minn, 1979, West Publishing, p 990.

7. *Robinson v. Jacksonville Shipyards,* 760 F. Supp. 1486 (Middle District of Florida, 1991).

8. Hays AS: Courts concede that the sexes think in unlike ways, *Wall Street Journal* B1, B5, May 28, 1991.

9. Struckman-Johnson CS, Struckman-Johnson D: Men's reactions to hypothetical female sexual advances, *Sex Roles* 1:387, 1994.

10. *Ellison v. Brady,* 924 F.2d 871 (9th Circuit 1991).

11. Naval Personnel Bulletin 15620: *Resolving conflict: following the light of personal behavior,* Washington, DC, 1993, US Government Printing Office.

12. *Disclosure,* 1995, Warner Bros.

13. Plevan BB, Borg JA: Expanded employer liability for supervisors' conduct in hostile work environments, *The National Law Journal* B5-B10, Aug 8, 1994.

14. Kruger P: See no evil, *Working Woman* 32-35, 64, 77, Jun 1995.

15. Graf LA, Hemmasi M: Risque humor: how it really affects the workplace, *HR Magazine* 64-69, Nov 1995.

16. Niven D: The case of hidden harassment, *Harvard Business Review* 12-27, Mar/Apr 1992. The scenario presented in this case study involves a female office worker who is sexually harassed by her supervisor's superior. The victim's supervisor learns of the sexual harassment by chance, and, when questioned about it, the victim does not want it to be reported. The case analysis offers the opinions of several human resource management and legal experts on how the victim's immediate supervisor should proceed.

17. Lopez JA: Control the damage of a false accusation of sexual harassment, *Wall Street Journal* B1, Jan 12, 1994.

18. *Oncale v. Sundowner Offshore Services, Inc* (96-586, reported in Felenthal E. High Court to rule on whether law bars same-sex harassment), *Wall Street Journal* B12, Jun 10, 1997.

19. *Oncale v. Sundowner Offshore Services, Inc,* 83 F.3d 118 (5th ca 1996).

20. *Quick v. Donaldson Company, Inc,* 90 F.3d 1372 (8th ca 1996).

21. Title IX of the Education Amendments of 1972, 20 United States Code Sections 1681-1683.

22. deMayo RA: Patient sexual behaviors and sexual harassment: a national survey of physical therapists, *Physical Therapy* 77:739, 1997.

23. *Oslund v. United States,* Civ. No. 4-88-323 (US District Court, District of Minnesota, Oct 23, 1989).

Suggested Readings

American Speech-Language-Hearing Association: *Gender issues and health: compensation and gender,* Rockville, Md, 1995, The Association.

American Physical Therapy Association: *Gender issues in employment under federal law: an American physical therapy white paper,* Alexandria, Va, 1995, APTA.

Black's law dictionary, ed 3, St Paul, Minn, 1979, West Publishing, p 990.

deMayo RA: Patient sexual behaviors and sexual harassment: a national survey of physical therapists, *Physical Therapy* 77:739, 1997.

Ellison v. Brady, 924 F.2d 871 (9th Circuit 1991).

Equal Employment Opportunity Commission: *Sex discrimination guidelines,* EEOC 29 Code of Federal Regulations 1604.11, Federal Register, 45:74677, 1980.

Felenthal E: High court to rule on whether law bars same-sex harassment, *Wall Street Journal* B12, Jun 10, 1997.

Graf LA, Hemmasi M: Risque humor: how it really affects the workplace, *HR Magazine* 64-69, Nov 1995.

Hays AS: Courts concede that the sexes think in unlike ways, *Wall Street Journal* B1, B5, May 28, 1991.

Kruger P: See no evil, *Working Woman* 32-35, 64, 77, Jun 1995.

Lopez JA: Control the damage of a false accusation of sexual harassment, *Wall Street Journal* B1, Jan 12, 1994.

Magretta J: Will She Fit In? *Harvard Business Review* 75(2):18, 1997.

Niven D: The case of hidden harassment, *Harvard Business Review* 12-27, Mar/Apr 1992.

Plevan BB, Borg JA: Expanded employer liability for supervisors' conduct in hostile work environments, *The National Law Journal* B5-B10, Aug 8, 1994.

Purtilo R: *Health professional and patient interaction,* ed 4, Philadelphia, 1990, WB Saunders, p 149.

Naval Personnel Bulletin 15620: *Resolving conflict: following the light of personal behavior,* Washington, DC, 1993, US Government Printing Office.

Robinson v. Jacksonville Shipyards, 760 F. Supp. 1486 (Middle District of Florida, 1991).

Scott RW: Sexual misconduct, *PT Magazine of Physical Therapy* 1(1)L78, 1993.

Stromber CD, Haggarty DJ, Leibenluft RF, et al: Physical contact and sexual relations with patients. In *The psychologist's legal handbook,* Washington, DC, 1988, Council for National Register of Health Service Providers in Psychology.

Struckman-Johnson CS, Struckman-Johnson D: Men's reactions to hypothetical female sexual advances, *Sex Roles* 1:387, 1994.

Title VII of the Civil Rights Act of 1964, 42 United States Code Section 2000e-16.

Title IX of the Education Amendments of 1972, 20 United States Code Sections 1681-1683.

Life and Death Decision Making

This chapter addresses ethical and legal issues involving the extremes of life. The chapter begins with discussion of passive and active euthanasia. Next, patient capacity is explored, followed by analysis of "do-not-resuscitate" orders. The chapter next overviews the federal Patient Self-Determination Act of 1990 and the two principal types of patient advance directives, living wills, and durable powers of attorney for health care. Discussion follows on the issue of a federal constitutional (privacy) right to die, with or without physician assistance. The chapter concludes with discussion of cloning.

●

Rehabilitation professionals work intensively with patients who are at or may be near the end of their lives. As rehabilitation team members, these professionals actively participate in conferences in which life and death issues involving their patients are addressed. Although none of the representative professional ethics codes (i.e., codes for occupational and physical therapy, and for orthotics and prosthetics) directly address professional responsibilities related to patient life and death decision making, all of these ethics codes indirectly address such issues through provisions requiring professionals to respect patient autonomy,[1] maintain patient confidentiality,[2] and act with beneficence toward patients under their care,[3] among numerous other issues.

Life and death decisions are largely made by patients (or their surrogate decision makers) and their primary physicians and surgeons. Rehabilitation professionals have the opportunity to offer unique insight about patients under their care to surrogate and physician decision makers, as members of institutional ethics committees, as primary rehabilitation team members, and in other important capacities.

This chapter provides an overview of important mixed law–professional ethical problems, issues, and dilemmas concerning life and death decision making.

Euthanasia

The Greek word **euthanasia** signifies "good" or "easy death." No area of health care professional service delivery has generated greater confusion, controversy, or judicial oversight than the area of euthanasia. Euthanasia seemingly involves conflicts among, and inconsistent compliance on the part of health care providers with, the four biomedical ethical principles of autonomy, beneficence, nonmaleficence, and justice. Is any form of euthanasia ethically, legally, and/or morally acceptable?

Euthanasia issues most often (but not always) center around patients who are either terminally ill or in a persistent vegetative state. A **terminally ill** patient is one with an incurable disease that is expected to result in the patient's death.[4] A patient who is in a **persistent vegetative state** is one who may exhibit "motor reflexes, but evinces no indication of significant cognitive function."[5] Classifying a patient as either terminally ill or in a persistent vegetative state has not only medical significance, it has legal, ethical, economic, and sociocultural implications as well.[6]

Processes such as the withdrawal or withholding of ordinary or extraordinary life-sustaining support devices or measures, or of sustenance, represent means of **passive euthanasia. Active euthanasia,** on the other hand, involves deliberate intervention by health care providers or others that facilitate or cause patients' demise. Although the United States Supreme Court in essence legitimized passive euthanasia in its 1990 *Cruzan*[7] decision (discussed in greater detail in this chapter),

How can health care professionals honor patients' or surrogates' wishes concerning continuation or discontinuation of treatment or other care measures in ways that evidence respect for patient autonomy and yet not violate the duty to "do harm" to these patients?

neither the states nor the federal government has sanctioned active euthanasia as legally and ethically acceptable medical practice.

On November 8, 1994, the voters in Oregon passed initiative Measure 16, also called the Oregon Death with Dignity Act (ODDA), which is the nation's first physician-assisted suicide law. ODDA authorizes physicians to write prescriptions for competent, terminally ill adult patients who are expected to die within 6 months, when such patients meet statutory requirements, including the making of three separate requests for suicide, obtaining a second medical opinion concerning their prognosis, and complying with the requisite 15-day waiting period.[8]

The law excludes from coverage (1) those competent adult patients physically unable to take the lethal medication on their own; (2) patients with non-terminal diagnoses, including chronic, debilitating conditions; (3) execution of patient requests for suicide made through advance directives or surrogate decision makers; and (4) non-Oregonians.[9] The ODDA does not compel physicians and other health care professionals to take part in assisting patients to die. The law has never been implemented because of a temporary federal court injunction. In November 1997, Oregon voters rejected reconsideration of ODDA.[10]

Withdrawing and Withholding of Care

Competent versus Incompetent Patients

Patient competency, or **capacity,** is an issue that is critically important to health care professionals, attorneys, and jurists, who may act in ways (or sanction such action) that result in cessation of patients' lives based on a competency determination. Whereas health care professionals are expected to respect the autonomous right of competent patients to make decisions regarding their care and lives during periods of incapacitation, the legal standards for decisional mental capacity are varied and ambiguous.

Such standards include, among others, the Hopkins Competency Assessment Test (HCAT), which scores a patient's comprehension of informed consent disclosure information imparted in the form of an essay (read to the patient at three different reading comprehension levels—sixth grade, eighth grade, and first-year collegiate) by a physician or other primary health care professional. A patient can score between zero and ten on the test; a score of four or greater evidences capacity, whereas a score of less than four indicates patient incapacity to make health care decisions.[11]

Some authorities urge health care professionals to develop relevant clinical standards for health care decision making, based on scientific evidence such as outcomes data that allow for flexibility to fit each patient's situation and needs, rather than using any rigid "capacimeter" based on traditional or nontraditional competency standards.[12]

Do Not Resuscitate Orders

Do not resuscitate (DNR) orders in patient medical records are written physician directives to staff health care professionals that preclude the otherwise automatic initiation of cardiopulmonary resuscitation (CPR) efforts in the event of patient cardiorespiratory arrest. DNR orders do not affect other life-sustaining interventions.

There are four principal circumstances that may justify the writing of a DNR order. They are:

- At the request of a competent patient
- Pursuant to a valid patient request under a living will or similar legal instrument
- At the request of a properly designated third-party surrogate decision maker empowered under a durable power of attorney for health care decision making
- When, in the judgment of a patient's primary physician (and another, or other, physicians as required by law or institutional policy), resuscitative efforts would be futile.[13]

Health care providers must learn (and take the time) to communicate more effectively with patients regarding patients' desires on end-of-life care. A recent Robert Wood Johnson Foundation study revealed that in 47 percent of cases, physicians were unaware that patients under their care did not want CPR in the event of cardiac arrest.[14] Since managed care has limited the amount of time physicians, in particular, can spend with individual patients, nonphysician rehabilitation professionals who are able to spend more quality time with patients can help physicians and patients by expeditiously communicating patient expressions of desires concerning treatment options to the patients' primary physicians and to the rest of the rehabilitation team.

Primary physicians must carefully document specific information concerning DNRs in patients' medical records. Although the requisite information varies from state to state, the following information is commonly required to be annotated:

- Justification and supporting rationale for the DNR order
- Information on a DNR-patient's condition, mental capacity, and advance directives
- Summary of physician communications with the patient and/or the patient's significant others, guardian, or surrogate decision maker
- Summary of input from an institutional ethics committee or other ethics consultants[15]

Impact of the Patient Self-Determination Act of 1990

The Patient Self-Determination Act of 1990 (PSDA),[16] introduced by Senator John Danforth of Missouri, is a federal statute that codifies patients' right to control treat-

> Since managed care has limited the amount of time physicians can spend with individual patients, nonphysician rehabilitation professionals who are able to spend more quality time with patients can help physicians and patients by expeditiously communicating patient expressions of desires concerning treatment options.

ment-related decisions, both routine and extraordinary.[17] The PSDA obligates hospitals, HMOs, long-term care facilities, home health agencies, hospices, and other health care organizations receiving Medicare and Medicaid funds to its provisions.

Fundamental purposes of the PSDA include (1) educating patients about their rights to formulate **advance directives;** (2) increasing the number of advance directives executed by patients; (3) facilitating compliance, on the part of physicians and allied health professionals, with patients' wishes concerning life-sustaining medical interventions; and (4) addressing, through advance directives, the high costs of end-of-life medical care.

Advance directives are legal instruments that memorialize a patient's desires concerning life-sustaining measures to be undertaken in the event of the patient's incapacitation, which a patient executes while legally competent. Common varieties of advance directives include living wills and durable powers of attorney for health care decisions.

A **living will** is a legal document, signed by a patient, which states the patient's wishes concerning life-sustaining measures to be undertaken in the event of the patient's subsequent incompetence. A living will is also known as a *directive to physicians.* Statutory *natural death acts* are forms of living wills in effect in at least 33 states.[18] Most states require that a patient be both legally incompetent and terminally ill in order for a living will to become operative. Some states allow a living will to become operative when a patient is in a persistent vegetative state.

A **durable power of attorney for health care decisions,** a special power of attorney, is a legal document signed by a patient, which delegates health care decision making to an agent of the patient's choice. The power becomes operative upon the patient's legal incompetence to make such decisions for himself or herself. The patient normally may designate anyone—spouse, relative, friend, attorney, or other trusted person—as the surrogate health care decision maker.

Under the Texas Consent to Medical Treatment Act,[19] absent valid patient advance directives, the following relatives and other persons in descending order of priority are empowered to consent to medical treatment for incapacitated hospitalized inpatients or nursing home residents:

- Spouse
- Adult child as sole decision maker (with the consent of all other adult children)
- Majority of reasonably available adult children
- Parent(s)
- Another surrogate decision maker clearly identified by the patient
- Nearest living relative
- Clergy

The principle premise underlying the PSDA is respect for a patient's inherent right to self-determination and control over treatment decision making. A health care provider must, according to this premise, disclose to a patient sufficient information about a proposed course of treatment (i.e., the nature of the recommended intervention; its material risks, if any; reasonable alternatives to the proposed intervention; and expected benefits of treatment) to empower the patient to analyze the options and make an informed choice about whether to undergo or reject treatment.

The PSDA does not create any new substantive patient rights. Instead, it imposes affirmative procedural obligations on health care providers and facilities to whom the law applies. Among other requirements, the PSDA requires providers and facilities to:

- Provide written information to patients concerning their rights under state law to give informed consent or refusal of treatment and to make advance directives
- Provide patients with copies of institutional policies concerning informed patient decision making and advance directives
- Document in patient records whether or not patients have executed advance directives concerning treatment[20]

The Audie L. Murphy Memorial Veterans Hospital's policy statement on withholding and withdrawal of life support includes policies, procedures, and health professional responsibilities regarding patient advance directives. This policy statement, which also includes formats for a living will and a durable power of attorney for health care and patient treatment preferences, is an excellent model. It is reprinted in Appendix A.

Larsen and Eaton[21] did an exhaustive investigative analysis of the PSDA and reported that the law has enjoyed only limited success since its enactment. The reasons for its limited success include the facts that many patients are unaware of their right to make enforceable advance directives, many patients are unwilling to execute advance directives, and physicians either do not know of or fail to comply with valid patient advance directives.

Drs. Carney and Morrison[22] urge physicians to communicate more effectively with patients about their patients' wishes concerning end-of-life treatment decisions. To aid physicians and other health care professionals in learning about their patients' values and desires, the Center for Health Law and Ethics of the University of New Mexico School of Law's Institute of Public Policy developed a Values History Form,[23] which patients can easily complete in about 10 minutes. The Values History Form is reprinted in Appendix B. Its authors graciously did not copyright the form and urge health professional readers to use and/or modify it for their particular needs.

Many patients are unaware of their right to make enforceable advance directives. Many patients are unwilling to execute advance directives. Physicians either do not know of or fail to comply with valid patient advance directives.

151

Is There a "Constitutional Right to Die?"

The mixed legal-ethical issue of whether there is a legal right to die under the federal constitution has baffled jurists, attorneys, politicians, and health care professionals and policy makers for some time. In a society like ours that is so acutely legalistic, this issue seemingly has taken on a life of its own (no pun intended).

The United States Supreme Court has confronted this issue in three cases: *Cruzan v. Director, Missouri Department of Health*,[24] and, decided on the same day, *Washington v. Glucksberg*[25] and *Vacco v. Quill*.[26] In all three cases, the Supreme Court declined to interpret the existence of a federal constitutional right to die.

On January 11, 1983, Nancy Beth Cruzan was involved in a roll-over motor vehicle accident, in which she suffered anoxia for up to 14 minutes, eventually leaving her in a persistent vegetative state. After 4 years, her parents sought judicial permission of the Missouri state courts to remove Nancy's artificial feeding and hydration tubes, so that she could die naturally. Nancy, like most Americans, had not executed any advance directives. The Missouri Supreme Court overturned the ruling of the trial-level court granting the Cruzans' permission to remove Nancy's nutritional apparatus, finding that such action could only take place if there was clear and convincing evidence that this action comported with Nancy's wishes.

The United States Supreme Court affirmed the decision of the Missouri Supreme Court and held that (1) there is a federal constitutional (privacy) right to refuse medical treatment, which survives a patient's subsequent incapacity, and (2) it is the states' prerogative to determine the legal standard for establishing an incompetent patient's wishes concerning life-sustaining treatment. States establish such procedural safeguards on behalf of incapacitated patients under their inherent *parens patriae* power.

In June 1997, in *Washington v. Glucksberg* and *Vacco v. Quill*, the United States Supreme Court upheld two state statutes (Washington and New York) banning physician-assisted suicide, a form of active euthanasia. The Court found that there is no fundamental federal constitutional privacy right to unregulated assisted suicide. Five of the nine Supreme Court justices left open, in their separate concurring opinions, the possibility of revisiting the issue of assisted suicide at some later time.

Cloning

Another salient bioethics issue involves cloning. Cloning is the process of reproducing a genetically identical duplicate of an organism. This issue became critical early in 1997 when Scottish researchers cloned a sheep and sought a patent for their cloning process. (The United States Supreme Court previously ruled that living organisms are potentially patentable.)

There are few legal impediments to cloning.[27] One prominent legal prohibition is the federal research funding ban on human embryo research, which includes cloning. At the time of the writing of this book, the eighteen-member National Bioethics Advisory Committee had recently reported that human cloning is immoral and unethical. However, the Commission seemed to sanction animal and human DNA and cell cloning.[28]

Summary

At the extremes of life, neither cloning nor assisted suicide is a constitutionally protected activity. In *Cruzan v. Director, Missouri Department of Health,* however, the United States Supreme Court did recognize a fundamental right in patients to refuse medical treatment and end-of-life interventions such as nutrition and hydration. Although passive euthanasia is sanctioned as legally and ethically acceptable, no state (except Oregon) allows physicians or others to actively assist patients to commit suicide. Jack Kevorkian stubbornly refuses to accept this fact, as he assists patient after patient to "end their suffering."

Rehabilitation professionals have a key role in educating patients about their rights to execute advance directives and have them respected by health care providers, and in reporting patient assertions of their wishes regarding life-sustaining measures to decision makers.

Cases and Questions

1. A 54-year-old terminally ill cancer patient expresses during an evaluation by an orthotist her desire to "die with dignity." What action(s), if any, should the orthotist take, based on the patient's assertion?

2. Review and carefully complete the "Values History Form" found in Appendix B. Based on your answers, what have you learned about your personal values regarding life and independence?

Suggested Answers for Cases and Questions

1. Analyze this problem under the **systems approach** to health professional ethical decision making.

Step 1: **Identify the ethical problem.** The patient has made a statement during orthotic evaluation, which possibly impacts on end-of-life medical interventions. The patient has the inherent right to self-determination over health care interventions affecting her person and body. What action(s), if any, should the orthotist take, based on the patient's assertion?

continued

Suggested Answers for Cases and Questions—cont'd

Step 2: **Identify relevant facts and unknowns; formulate reasonable assumptions.** *Facts:* The patient is terminally ill with cancer; she is undergoing orthotic evaluation; she has expressed a desire to "die with dignity." *Unknowns:* Family situation, advance directives in force, other considerations? *Assumptions:* The patient appears competent and sincere and in need of professional consultation regarding her statement.

Step 3: **Assess viable courses of action.** (1) Take no action, because the patient's statement is confidential. (2) Document the patient's statement, but take no further action. (3) Alert the patient's physician and nurse about her statement.

Step 4: **Implement a course of action.** Execute option 3—alert the patient's physician and nurse.

Step 5: **Obtain feedback on the chosen course of action; modify or change, as necessary.** The orthotist should follow up the next day with the physician or nurse regarding action taken based on the patient's reported statement.

2. Your answers to the questions posed may lead you to execute one or more advance directives concerning your own end-of-life medical care. Please consult with your personal attorney for advice in drafting and executing such legal instruments. For those who do not have a personal attorney, attorney specialists are available at no cost or at nominal cost as a public service through the local county or parish bar association lawyer referral service.

References

1. American Occupational Therapy Association: *Occupational therapy code of ethics, principle 2 (autonomy, privacy, confidentiality)*, (Occupational therapy personnel shall respect the rights of the recipients of their services), Bethesda, Md, 1994, AOTA.

2. American Physical Therapy Association: *Guide for professional conduct, section 1.2, (confidential information)*, Alexandria, Va, 1997, APTA. (See also American Physical Therapy Association: *Guide for conduct of the affiliate member, section 2.3 [Protection of Privacy]*, Alexandria, Va, 1997, APTA.)

3. American Board for Certification in Orthotics and Prosthetics: *Canons of ethical conduct, canon 2.2 (orthosis and prosthesis evaluation and recommendation)*, Alexandria, Va, 1994, ABC.

4. Audie L. Murphy Memorial Veterans Hospital: *Policy memorandum no. 119617: withholding or withdrawal of life-sustaining treatment*, San Antonio, Tex, 1996, The Hospital.

5. *Cruzan v. Director, Missouri Department of Health*, 497 US 261 (1990).

6. Furrow BR, Johnson SH, Jost TS, Schwartz RL: *Health law: cases, materials and problems*, ed 2, St Paul, Minn, 1991, West Publishing, p 1056.

7. *Cruzan*, note 5.

8. Schuyler N: Helping the grim reaper, *California Lawyer* 33-35, Mar 1995.

9. Alpers A, Lo B: Physician-assisted suicide in Oregon: a bold experiment, *JAMA* 274:483, 1995.

10. Supreme Court refuses to hear challenge to Oregon's assisted suicide loaw, *Health Lawyers News,* Nov, 1997, pp 27-28.

11. Wolfe LM: A clarification of the standard of mental capacity in North Carolina for legal transactions of the elderly, *Wake Forest Law Review* 32(2):563, 1997.

12. Kapp MB, Mossan D: Measuring decisional capacity: cautions on the construction of a capacimeter, *Psychology, Public Policy, and Law* 2(1):73, 1996.

13. American Medical Association: Guidelines for the appropriate use of do not resuscitate orders: council on ethical and judicial affairs, *JAMA* 265:1868, 1991.

14. Patient's wishes on "end-of-life care" should be discussed with health professionals, *PT Bulletin* 19, Dec 22, 1995.

15. Woodruff WA: Letting life run its course: do-not-resuscitate orders and withdrawal of life-sustaining treatment, *Army Lawyer* 6-18, Apr, 1989.

16. *The Patient Self-Determination Act of 1990,* 42 United States Code Sections 1395cc and 1396a.

17. Scott RW: Guaranteeing patient rights: it's the law, *Advance for Directors in Rehab* 43-44, Sep/Oct, 1992.

18. Texas Natural Death Act, Acts 1989, 71st Legislature, ch 672 (Historical and Statutory Notes: Comparative Laws).

19. Texas Consent to Medical Treatment Act, Acts 1993, 73rd Legislature, ch 313.

20. Patient Self-Determination Act, Section 1395cc(f).

21. Larsen EJ, Eaton TA: The limits of advance directives: a history and assessment of the patient self-determination act, *Wake Forest Law Review* 32(2):249, 1997.

22. Carney MT, Morrison RS: Advance directives: when, why, and how to start talking, *Geriatrics* 52(4):65, 1997.

23. Center for Health Law and Ethics, Institute of Public Law: *Values history form,* Albuquerque, NM, 1993, University of New Mexico School of Law.

24. See note 5.

25. Individual rights, *Health Law Digest* 25(7):41, 1997.

26. *Ibid,* p 42.

27. Jacobs MA, Davis A: Cloning faces few legal barriers for now, *Wall Street Journal* B6, Feb 25, 1997.

28. Friend T: Bioethics study: no human clones, *USA Today* 1A, Jun 6, 1997.

Suggested Readings

Alpers A, Lo B: Physician-assisted suicide in Oregon: a bold experiment, *JAMA* 274:483, 1995.

American Medical Association: Guidelines for the appropriate use of do not resuscitate orders: council on ethical and judicial affairs, *JAMA* 265:1868, 1991.

Beaubien G, Roder D: Fighting to die: assisted deaths/DNRs still pose medical/ethical dilemmas to physicians, *San Antonio Medical Gazette* 22-23, Oct. 10-16, 1996.

Capron, AM: Constitutionalizing death, *Hastings Center Report* 23-24, Nov-Dec, 1995.

Capron AM: Sledding in Oregon, *Hastings Center Report* 34-35, Jan-Feb, 1995.

Carney MT, Morrison RS: Advance directives: when, why, and how to start talking, *Geriatrics* 52(4):65, 1997.

Center for Health Law and Ethics, Institute of Public Law: *Values history form,* Albuquerque, NM, 1993, University of New Mexico School of Law.

Cruzan v. Director, Missouri Department of Health, 497 US 261 (1990).

Emanuel EJ: The painful truth about euthanasia, *Wall Street Journal* A18, Jan 7, 1997.

Emanuel EJ, Emanuel LL: Proxy decision making for incompetent patients, *JAMA* 267:2067, 1992.

Felder M: We want you to pull the plug, *Medical Economics* 115-118, Jun 24, 1996.

Friend T: Bioethics study: no human clones, *USA Today* 1A, Jun 6, 1997.

Furrow BR, Johnson SH, Jost TS, Schwartz RL: *Health law: cases, materials and problems,* ed 2, St Paul, Minn, 1991, West Publishing, p 1056.

Individual rights, *Health Law Digest* 25(7):41, 1997.

Jacobs MA, Davis A: Cloning faces few legal barriers for now, *Wall Street Journal* B6, Feb 25, 1997.

Kapp MB, Mossan D: Measuring decisional capacity: cautions on the construction of a capacimeter, *Psychology, Public Policy, and Law* 2(1):73, 1996.

Kleyman P: Assisted suicide debate sent to states, *Aging Today* 18(4):1,3, 1997.

Larsen EJ, Eaton TA: The limits of advance directives: a history and assessment of the patient self-determination act, *Wake Forest Law Review* 32(2):249, 1997.

Luce JM: Ethical principles in critical care, *JAMA* 263:696, 1990.

Mauro T: Assisted suicide ban upheld, *USA Today* 1A, 4A, Jun 27-29, 1997.

McCartney RD: May you never be put in this position, *Medical Economics* 95-98, Jul 15, 1996.

McClung JA, Kamer RS: Legislating ethics: implications of New York's do-not-resuscitate law, *N Engl J Med* 323:270, 1990.

Orentlicher D: The legalization of physician-assisted suicide, *N Engl J Med* 335:663, 1996.

Orentlicher D: The right to die after Cruzan, *JAMA* 264:2444, 1990.

Patient's wishes on "end-of-life care" should be discussed with health professionals, *PT Bulletin* 19, Dec 22, 1995.

The Patient Self-Determination Act of 1990, 42 United States Code Sections 1395cc and 1396a.

Primono MP: Palliative care is the real focus of end-of-life medicine, *ACP Observer* 16(7):2, 1996.

Schlomann P: Ethical decision making in a neonatal intensive care unit: the nurse's role, *Neonatal Intensive Care* 44-47, 53-54, Jul/Aug, 1996.

Schuyler N: Helping the grim reaper, *California Lawyer* 33-35, Mar 1995.

Scott RW: Guaranteeing patient rights: it's the law, *Advance for Directors in Rehab* 43-44, Sep/Oct, 1992.

Smedira NG, Evans BH, Grais LS, et al: Withholding and withdrawal of life support from the critically ill, *N Engl J Med* 322:309, 1990.

Wolfe LM: A clarification of the standard of mental capacity in North Carolina for legal transactions of the elderly, *Wake Forest Law Review* 32(2):563, 1997.

Woodruff WA: Letting life run its course: do-not-resuscitate orders and withdrawal of life-sustaining treatment, *Army Lawyer* 6-18, Apr, 1989.

Professional Ethics in Research, Education, and Patient Care Delivery

This chapter examines selected health professional ethical concerns in research, education, and clinical practice. Research issues are addressed first, including the requirements for subject protection from harm and informed consent. Discussion of educational setting ethical concerns follows. Academicians, clinical faculty and guest lecturers, and health professional students all have defined ethical duties incident to the educational process. Ethics committees and consultations and managed care ethical issues are addressed next. The chapter concludes with discussion of ethical and legal duties of health care professionals to report abuse and other events to authorities.

•

Ethical Issues in Human Subjects Research

Ethical issues in research settings center largely on two issues: the protection of human research subjects and the integrity of research processes.[1] Federal regulations governing the use of human subjects in research promulgated by the Department of Health and Human Services[2] are derived, in part, from United States law and, in part, from customary international law and multinational human rights treaties. Responsibility for the protection of human research subjects rests with institutional review boards (IRBs), which are multidisciplinary committees that establish research protocol guidelines; review and approve research proposals for their institutions that involve human research subjects; and enforce compliance with federal, state, and institutional requirements and standards.

The integrity of research scientists is a paramount concern to the research community, for obvious reasons. From the funding of research projects to public trust, research—especially involving human subjects—must have the respect of the scientific community, government, and public-at-large.

Researchers, similar to health care clinicians, academicians, and students, have ethical responsibilities. Scientists have the same core values that others have within a given profession[3] and are obligated to comply with the professional codes of ethics governing their respective disciplines.

Researchers are ethically bound to protect the well-being of research subjects and to ensure that each individual is provided detailed disclosure of information regarding the research, ensuring that informed consent is given to participate. They must also maintain appropriate confidentiality of the personal identities of research subjects. Researchers must avoid conflicts of interest that might bias their research findings. They are similarly obliged to avoid distorting or misrepresenting results, and they must appropriately credit others for their source materials and contributions to research projects.[4]

The representative rehabilitation professional codes of ethics address research concerns. For example, Section 4.3 (Research) of the *Guide for Professional Conduct* of the American Physical Therapy Association reads:

> A. Physical therapists shall support research activities that contribute knowledge for improved patient care.
>
> B. Physical therapists engaged in research shall ensure:
>
> > 1. Consent of subjects;
> > 2. Confidentiality of the data on individual subjects and the personal identities of the subjects;
> > 3. Well-being of all subjects in compliance with facility regulations and the laws of the jurisdiction in which the research is conducted;

> Researchers are ethically bound to protect the well-being of research subjects and to ensure that each person is provided detailed disclosure of information regarding the research, ensuring that informed consent is given to participate.

4. Absence of fraud and plagiarism;

5. Full disclosure of support received;

6. Appropriate acknowledgment of individuals making a contribution to the research;

7. Assurance that animal subjects used in research are treated humanely and in compliance with facility regulations and laws of the jurisdiction in which the research experimentation is conducted.

C. Physical therapists shall report to appropriate authorities any acts in the conduct or presentation of research that appear unethical or illegal.

Principle 2D of the *Occupational Therapy Code of Ethics* reads in part:

Occupational therapy personnel shall respect the individual's right to refuse...involvement in research...activities.

Canon 3.3 of the *Canons of Ethical Conduct* of the American Board for Certification in Orthotics and Prosthetics (ABC) provides the most detailed, directive guidance regarding research activities as follows:

All orthotists and prosthetists *shall* [emphases added] support research activities that contribute to the understanding of improved patient care. In the event that any orthotist or prosthetist desires to engage in a research project or study, he or she shall first ensure that:

(i) All patients affiliated with such projects or studies consent in writing to the use of the results of the study;

(ii) Data and information regarding the patient remains confidential;

(iii) Well-being of the patient shall be the primary concern;

(iv) Research is conducted in accordance with all federal and state law;

(v) There is an absence of fraud;

(vi) All data is fully disclosed;

(vii) There is an appropriate acknowledgment of individuals making contribution to the research;

(viii) In the event that any acts in the conduct or presentation of research appear to be unethical or illegal, the orthotist or prosthetist shall *immediately* report the unethical or illegal conduct to ABC and, if appropriate, the applicable law enforcement authority [emphasis added].

159

Health Professional Student and Faculty Ethical Concerns

In professional education settings, academicians (including guest lecturers), clinical faculty, and students all have ethical responsibilities. The same fundamental duties of competency, confidentiality, fidelity, respect, and truth that apply to professional-patient relationships apply with equal force to relationships between students and faculty. Many of these professional ethical duties are codified into case law and statutes, making them legal duties as well. For example, the legal duty of confidentiality of student records incumbent on academicians and educational program administrators is governed by the Family Education Rights and Privacy Act of 1974 (the "Buckley Amendment").[5]

Students, as well as faculty, have fundamental professional ethical duties governing their conduct. For example, relative to truth, students have the ethical duties not to cheat on examinations and not to plagiarize or fail to credit, as appropriate, the work product of others when paraphrasing them. Health professional students also have the ethical duty not to intentionally defraud prospective employers by signing pre-employment contracts solely to receive current financial incentives.

Sanctions for violations of ethical duties in professional education exist along a progressive continuum, just as they do along the disciplinary continuum in employment settings. Students who violate ethical obligations may face the award of a failing grade, or suspension or expulsion from their educational programs for serious breaches of ethics. Faculty who breach professional ethical standards may incur the loss of a chance for tenure or even the loss of employment for serious breaches of their ethical responsibilities.

Faculty and student ethical responsibilities are commonly spelled out with varying degrees of clarity in faculty and student handbooks, respectively. Although standards may appear vague, sanctions for violations of standards cannot be stated in a vague fashion, because of the constitutional procedural due process considerations of notice and substantive fairness, which are prerequisites to adverse action—at least in public institutions of higher learning.

Among other ethical duties of academic and clinical faculty are the duty to certify that health professional students participating in clinical affiliations are competent to perform the tasks expected of them and the duty to supervise students in laboratory and clinical settings, as appropriate. Students bear the special ethical duties to follow reasonable instructions issued to them by their professors and clinical instructors and to act only within the scope of their personal and legal competence.

Ethics Committees and Consultations

Institutional ethics committees (IECs) are multidisciplinary committees within health care organizations, which include health care and related professionals (i.e., clergy,

The same fundamental duties of competency, confidentiality, fidelity, respect, and truth that apply to professional-patient relationships apply with equal force to relationships between students and faculty.

social workers, attorneys), and occasionally lay members. In addition to their educative and policy-making roles, IECs offer consultative services to physicians and other health care providers and administrations on cases involving ethical problems, issues, and dilemmas.

A primary goal of an IEC ethics consultation is to provide collective advice to physicians and other clinical health care decision makers about patient care issues. As the adage goes, "Two (or six, or twelve) heads are always better than one." The consultative role of the IEC to physicians and others is advisory, not directive. It remains, as it always has been, the primary responsibility of a patient's attending or primary physician or surgeon (or other primary care professional) to execute patient care decisions. Through IEC intervention, however, it is often easier for physicians and other health care providers and their patients and families to reach ethical consensus concerning optimal patient care decisions.

What is the role of an attorney in the ethics consultative process? A health care organization attorney should act as a legal consultant to an IEC, offering advice on the legal implications of alternative decisions to decision makers. An attorney should neither dictate a solution to the IEC nor be permitted to dominate discussion with risk management concerns.[6] Attorneys are educated by law schools to be legal advisors, not surrogate decision makers (although they are too often misused as such). An IEC (or any decision maker) should never have to say, "We're just doing what the lawyer told us to do."

Ethics consultations can be obtained from sources other than IECs as well. Private ethics consultants and professional associations are other sources for ethics consultation. By way of example, ETHICSearch is a service of the American Bar Association's Standing Committee on Ethical and Professional Responsibility for member attorneys, at no cost for routine matters or at nominal cost for complicated inquiries requiring consultant research.[7]

Managed Care and Health Care Professional Ethics

The advent of managed health care delivery in the 1980s and its exponential growth during the 1990s have resulted in both problems and promise for health care professionals. **Managed care** is an amorphous concept that has been defined in different ways by various authorities.[8,9,10] Everyone agrees, however, that managed care is a system of health care service delivery that focuses significant attention on cost containment, as well as the quality of patient care delivered by the system. Managed care in the 1990s has become the private sector analog to the failed federal public-sector health care reform initiatives of the early part of the decade.

Managed care has created profound challenges for professionals in all health care disciplines and for specialists within specific disciplines. Rehabilitation health care professionals, for example, find themselves being asked to assume ever-increasing responsibilities in multiple roles, such as multiskilled clinicians,[11] supervisors of increasing numbers and types of support and "extender" personnel, administrators, educators, researchers, and consultants,[12] among other possible roles.

Managed care has created significant ethical concerns, most of which are discussed throughout this book. Of principal concern is the fact that, for the first time, under managed care, the health care delivery system has made cost containment a co-equal (hopefully not a higher) consideration with optimal quality patient care delivery. As the health care delivery system has become more businesslike, *patients* have come to be known as *enrollees, plan participants,* and *subscribers,* among other euphemisms. Managed care has focused public attention on and intensified providers' conflicts of interest with their patients, because many providers feel compelled to "do more with less" and elect not to disclose treatment-related information to patients.

Patients have begun to question the efficacy of managed care. In expressing their concern about the quality of health care delivery, patients generally report satisfaction with traditional fee-for-service health care and dissatisfaction with managed care–model health care delivery systems.[13] Considerations of health professional ethics and concern for the integrity and status of health care demand that changes be made to the current health care paradigm, and they are occurring—through governmental intervention, public pressure, health care provider input, and other means.

> Managed care has created significant ethical concerns, one of which is the fact that, for the first time, the health care delivery system has made cost containment a co-equal consideration with optimal quality patient care delivery.

Reporting Requirements Incumbent On Rehabilitation Professionals

Rehabilitation health professionals and their assistants and extenders have the professional ethical and (in most states) the legal duty to identify and report suspected patient abuse to law enforcement authorities. Patient abuse categories reflect patient age or relational status to the abuser, as follows: child, domestic (spousal), and elder abuse.

Research study reports indicate that health care professionals do not report suspected abuse involving their patients as often as they are required,[14] even where nonreporting constitutes a criminal offense.[15] Reasons preferred for failing to report include lack of training on the signs and symptoms of abuse, overwork, and fear of defamation liability exposure, among others. Professional associations, such as the American Physical Therapy Association, offer guidelines for recognizing patient abuse.[16]

Patient abuse may be physical (including sexual) and psychological (including neglect). Common signs and symptoms of patient abuse include the following, among others:

- Reticence; failure to make eye contact
- Annoyance over personal questions during the taking of a patient history[17]
- Withdrawal from touch
- Untreated or unexplained injury
- Skin irritation, scratches, burns, lacerations, or bruising
- Malnutrition; dehydration
- Unexplained weight loss
- Pallor; sunken eyes and/or cheeks
- Poor hygiene
- Soiled clothes; clothing inappropriate for the season or setting
- Permitting a caregiver or other chaperone to answer questions for her or him

As a matter of professional ethical and legal duty and of prudent liability risk management, every health care clinical manager should ensure that all clinical health care providers receive periodic instruction and reinstruction by competent professionals on patient abuse. The act of reporting suspected patient abuse should not give rise to liability (although it might give rise to litigation), because health care providers are afforded **qualified,** or limited **immunity** from defamation liability for making good faith reports of suspected patient abuse to authorities.

Additional reporting requirements incumbent on health professionals include:

- Reporting infectious and occupational diseases to public health entities and OSHA, respectively
- Reporting gunshot and stab wounds to law enforcement authorities
- Reporting unsafe equipment to the product manufacturer and the Food and Drug Administration

Providers are encouraged to consult proactively with legal counsel regarding their state-and situation-specific reporting obligations.

Summary

Health professional obligations pervade the gambit of potential practice settings. In health care research—whether or not human subjects are involved—researchers have special professional ethical duties to be truthful and accurate and to acknowledge contributors and sources. In educational settings, academicians and clinical faculty owe a duty of professionalism to students, as well as the duties to instruct them appropriately to prepare them for entry-level practice and to accurately and fairly assess and report

163

their level of competence. Students, too, owe professional ethical duties of respect, fidelity, and candor, among traditional others. All health care professionals owe a special duty to be able to identify and report suspected child, domestic, and elder abuse in their patients.

Managed care has refocused health care delivery away from quality patient care exclusively toward a dual focus on patient care and cost containment. Managed care is fraught with ethical problems and issues and dilemmas, particularly involving patient and provider access to services and conflicts of interest involving providers, organizations, and patients. As the system evolves through managed care into twenty-first century "managed health," a refocusing on patient welfare will predominate.

Cases and Questions

1. A 41-year-old female patient who has been referred for evaluation for a right below-knee prosthesis informs her evaluating prosthetist that she is being physically abused by her live-in boyfriend. The patient asks the prosthetist to keep the revelation confidential. What action should the prosthetist take?

2. As an interdisciplinary rehabilitation team exercise, develop, in small groups of three to eight people of different disciplines, fact-based hypothetical scenarios for ethics consultations. Assign roles for group members to play, and present the role play scenarios to one another at in-service education sessions. Assign one member of the group to critique the role play and facilitate discussion.

Suggested Answers for Cases and Questions

1. Analyze this problem under the **systems approach** to health professional ethical decision making.

Step 1: **Identify the ethical problem.** The patient has made a statement during prosthetic evaluation, giving rise to a reasonable suspicion of possible physical abuse of the patient by her live-in boyfriend. The patient requests nondisclosure of this revelation by her prosthetist. What should the prosthetist do?

Step 2: **Identify relevant facts and unknowns; formulate reasonable assumptions.** *Facts:* The patient has sustained a right below-knee amputation and has presented for prosthetic evaluation. She shows no signs or symptoms of abuse. *Unknowns:* Domestic situation. Does she really want this information to be kept confidential? Can the health professional legally and ethically comply with the patient's request for confidentiality? *Assumptions:* The patient appears competent and sincere.

Suggested Answers for Cases and Questions—cont'd

Step 3: **Assess viable courses of action.** (1) Take no action, because the patient's statement is confidential; (2) document the patient's statement, but take no further action; (3) alert the patient's physician and/or referral source and social service regarding the patient's statement.

Step 4: **Implement a course of action.** Execute option 3—alert the patient's physician and social service.

Step 5: **Obtain feedback on the chosen course of action; modify or change, as necessary.** The prosthetist should follow-up the next day with the physician or social service official regarding action taken based on the patient's reported statement.

2. Consider writing your ethics consultation role play exercises and submitting them for publication and commentary.

References

1. Portney LG, Watkins MP: *Foundations of clinical research: applications to practice,* Norwalk, Conn, 1993, Appleton & Lange.

2. Title 45 Code of Federal Regulations, Part 46: *Protection of human subjects,* Washington, DC, 1983, Dept of Health and Human Services.

3. *On being a scientist: responsible conduct in research,* ed 2, 1995, Washington, DC, National Academy Press, p 6-8.

4. *Ibid,* p 8-18.

5. The Family Educational Rights and Privacy Act of 1974, 20 United States Code Section 1232 et seq.

6. Mathis RD: The roles of the law and the lawyer in clinical ethics. In *Health care ethics short course,* San Antonio, Tex, 1993, Brooke Army Medical Center.

7. Stein RA: Just call the ethics experts, *ABA Journal* 98, Mar 1997.

8. Olsen GG: The coming wave: PSNs, PHOs, and PCCOs, *Rehab Management* 101-102, Oct/Nov 1995.

9. Schunk C: Understanding managed care: a glossary of terminology, *GeriNotes* 3(1):20, 1995.

10. Werning SC: A primer on managed care, *Healthcare Trends & Transitions* 5(1):10-13, 26-28, 46. 1993.

11. Arthur PR: The restructuring of America's hospitals: acute orthopedic services, *PT: Magazine of Physical Therapy* 2(7):35, 1994.

12. Richardson JK: The challenging roles facing PTs, *Healthcare Trends & Transitions* 5(1):34, 1993.

13. Americans concerned about health care, *PT Bulletin* 11, Aug 1, 1997.

14. 40% of health professional admit not reporting abuse, *PT Bulletin* 6, 40, Feb 21, 1990.

15. Arispe R: It's the law: health professionals required to report abuse and neglect, *San Antonio Medical Gazette* 4, Oct 10-16, 1996.

16. American Physical Therapy Association: *Guidelines for recognizing and providing care for victims of domestic abuse,* Alexandria, Vir, 1997, APTA.

17. Kimmel D: Helping patients disclose abuse, *Advance for Physical Therapists* 4, May 12, 1997.

Suggested Readings

American Physical Therapy Association: *Guidelines for recognizing and providing care for victims of domestic abuse,* Alexandria, Vir, 1997, APTA.

Americans Concerned About Health Care, *PT Bulletin* 11, Aug 1, 1997.

Council on Ethical and Judicial Affairs: Ethical issues in managed care, *JAMA* 273:330, 1995.

Kane RA: The ethics of healthcare delivery to elders in a managed care environment, *Managed Care & Aging* 3(2):1-2, 8, 1996.

Kimmel D: Helping patients disclose abuse, *Advance for Physical Therapists* 4, May 12, 1997.

Olsen GG: The coming wave: PSNs, PHOs, and PCCOs, *Rehab Management* 101-102, Oct/Nov 1995.

On being a scientist: responsible conduct in research, ed 2, Washington, DC, 1995, National Academy Press.

Physicians and domestic violence, *JAMA* 267:3190, 1992.

Portney LG, Watkins MP: *Foundations of clinical research: applications to practice,* Norwalk, Conn, 1993, Appleton & Lange.

Richardson JK: The challenging roles facing PTs, *Healthcare Trends & Transitions* 5(1):34, 1993.

Salladay SA: Rehabilitation, ethics, and managed care, *Rehab Management* 38-40, Oct/Nov 1996.

Schunk C: Understanding managed care: a glossary of terminology, *GeriNotes* 3(1):20, 1995.

Stein RA: Just call the ethics experts, *ABA Journal* 98, Mar 1997.

The Family Educational Rights and Privacy Act of 1974, 20 United States Code Section 1232 et seq.

Title 45 Code of Federal Regulations, Part 46: Protection of Human Subjects, Washington DC, 1983, Dept of Health and Human Services.

Werning SC: A primer on managed care, *Healthcare Trends & Transitions* 5(1):10-13, 26-28, 46, 1993.

Wilford Hall Medical Center: *Elder abuse symposium,* San Antonio, Tex, 1994, The Center.

Epilogue: Future Directions in Health Care Professional Ethics

The future of health care professional ethics is highly dependent on whether health care service delivery retains its special status in society, or whether it comes to be viewed by the public, political and legal systems, patients, and health care professionals as just another ordinary business enterprise. If health care becomes just another business or industry, the traditionally high professional ethical standards governing practice may devolve into the same general business ethical standards generally governing commercial ventures.

Managed care has refocused public, political, and professional attention on the fact that health care resources—monetary, human, and capital—are finite. Managed care has also contributed to the accelerated commercialization of health care and to a defocusing on optimal quality patient care, perhaps in favor of what can be termed "minimally acceptable" patient care standards.

Although health care delivery that is minimally acceptable satisfies the legal standard of care, professional ethical standards—focused on patient welfare, like the traditional health care delivery system—require that providers "do the right thing," that is, provide the best possible care for patients. Health professional ethical standards have not changed significantly to accommodate the business of managed care.

Perhaps new managed care models, such as "provider-sponsored organizations," will help refocus health care intensively on the patient and away from other interests. Eventually, managed care, in its present form, will pass as the system evolves, ever cognizant of its undergirding professional ethical and legal framework.

Appendixes

Appendix A: Audie L. Murphy Memorial Veterans Hospital

Withholding or Withdrawal of Life-Sustaining Treatment

1. **Purpose:** Pursuant to the provisions of the Department of Veterans Affairs, Veterans Health Administration Manual M-2, Part 1, Chapter 31, this policy defines the protocols for withholding or withdrawal of life-sustaining treatment at the Audie L. Murphy Memorial Veterans Hospital (ALMMVH). This Medical Center recognizes that:

   a. The competent patient has the right to determine which treatment options he/she will accept or decline including withholding or withdrawal of life-sustaining treatments.

   b. Life-sustaining treatments may be withheld or withdrawn:
      (1) At the oral or written request of a competent patient;
      (2) As specified by a valid advance directive when a patient lacks decision-making capacity; or
      (3) At the request of the surrogate decision maker on behalf of an incompetent patient.

   c. Patient decision making concerning life-sustaining treatment and the execution of advance directives is subject to the usual Medical Center procedures for securing and documenting informed consent.

2. **Policy:**

   a. Life-sustaining treatment means medical care, procedures, or interventions, which when applied to a patient with a terminal illness, would have little or no effect on the underlying disease, injury, or condition, and which would serve only to delay the timing of death. This may include, but is not limited to, *resuscitation,* artificial nutrition and hydration, mechanical ventilation, and dialysis.

   b. Terminal illness refers to a debilitating condition, which is incurable and which can be expected to cause death. This includes conditions where death is imminent, as well as chronic and debilitating conditions from which there is no reasonable hope of recovery (e.g., persistent vegetative state).

   c. An advance directive is an oral or written statement made by a competent patient who states his or her preferences regarding medical treatments, including, but not limited to, life-sustaining treatments or who designates a surrogate decision maker who will make decisions regarding medical care in the event the patient is unable to do so. These include the VA Living Will (VA Form 10-0137a), Durable Power of Attorney for Health Care (DPAHC) (VA Form 10-0137b), Treatment Preferences (VA Form 10-0137c), or valid relevant State-authorized advance directives.

d. State-authorized advance directives will be honored in most circumstances.

(1) The document must be produced and must conform to the requirements of state law. District counsel may be consulted to determine the validity of any document. Contact either the Hospital Attorney (ext 5270 or pager 79-661) or the District Counsel, Houston Texas (FTS 700-526-2352).

(2) To implement the document, the patient must lack decision-making capacity and have little or no likelihood of regaining it within a reasonable period of time as medically determined.

(3) The patient's wishes, as expressed in the document, will be followed as long as they do not conflict with usual Veterans Health Administration (VA) practices and procedures.

(4) If a non-VA advance directive is not valid under state law but is sufficient to constitute a valid VA advance directive, it will be followed.

(5) Deficient, nonbinding advance directives may serve as evidence of the patient's desires and may be used by the surrogate decision maker in making decisions.

e. Patients may designate a surrogate decision maker to direct the course of their medical treatment in the event they lose decision-making capacity. Patients will be encouraged to complete VA DPAHC forms but valid state-authorized DPAHC forms will also be accepted using the criteria listed above.

f. Patients may execute a Treatment Preferences form in addition to a Living Will and/or DPAHC.

g. Patients are not required to execute an advance directive as a condition to receiving care.

3. **Procedures:**

a. On admission to a VA facility, all patients will be asked by the *admission clerk,* if they possess an advance directive (Living Will, DPAHC, Treatment Preferences). This will be documented by answering "yes" or "no" on the attached form or on the computerized admission form (when available). If the patient does not possess an advance directive, appropriate written information explaining the patient's rights under Chapter 31 will be provided at this time.

(1) If they have previously filled out a VA advance directive, the unit clerk will move it forward in the consolidated health record to the current admission. The *unit clerk* will assure that all charts containing advance directives display on the outside "ADVANCE DIRECTIVE INSIDE" on VA form 10-1079, "Emergency Medical Identification," or other appropriate label.

(2) If the patient has a VA or non-VA advance directive, which has not previously been placed in his or her medical record, a copy of the document will be requested and placed in the medical record by the *unit clerk* who will also label the outside of the chart as above.

171

b.   The *nurse* who admits the patient will assure that the patient has indeed received the appropriate written information on admission if an advance directive has not been previously completed. The *nurse* will ask the patient if he or she desires to execute an advance directive and will notify the treating physician if the patient does not desire to do so. The *nurse* will document this activity in his or her notes.

c.   The treating physician has the responsibility to provide all necessary medical information to the patient who wishes to execute an advance directive and to be ready to answer any additional medical questions including explanation of medical terms in the Living Will and/or Treatment Preferences form prior to its execution.

   (1) VA procedures applicable to other forms of patient decision making, including those that govern physician-patient dialogue, and the security and documentation of inform consent apply equally to patient decision making concerning life-sustaining treatment.

   (2) With respect to patient decision making concerning life-sustaining treatment, the treating physician must document in the progress notes the patient's diagnosis and prognosis, an assessment of the patient's decision-making capacity, treatment options presented to the patient for consideration, and the patient's decisions regarding life-sustaining treatment.

   (3) When life-sustaining treatment is not in accord with prevailing medical practice (e.g., is futile), it need not be presented as a treatment option.

   (4) If the patient expresses a desire to prepare an advance directive, it will be documented by the treating physician or his or her clinical designee in the progress notes and a referral will be made to the *social work service*.

d.   The social worker will be knowledgeable about advance directives and will be able to educate the patient regarding the types of advance directives. The *social worker* will be ready to counsel the patient and his or her family regarding the implications of advance directives. While assisting the patient in the execution of the document, the *social worker* will assure that the patient has had all questions resolved by the appropriate disciplines. To aid in executing the advance directive the *social worker* will:

   (1) Assure that the advance directive conforms to the VA forms, which may include supplemental instructions if the patient wishes.

   (2) Have two witnesses sign the executed document who:

      (a) are not related to the patient by blood or marriage;

      (b) do not have financial interest in the patient's estate;

      (c) are not financially responsible for the patient;

      (d) may be employees of the social work service, chaplain service, or non-clinical VA employees if no other witnesses are available. The unavailability of other witnesses should be documented in a progress note.

(3) Give the original document to the patient.

(4) Provide copies of the document to the ward clerk for placement in the medical record. The unit clerk will also label the outside of the chart as described and enter the appropriate data into the patient's computer file.

(5) Provide a copy to the patient to give the surrogate decision maker.

(6) Indicate in the progress notes that an advance directive has been executed and notify the treatment team.

e. Other services such as the *Chaplain Service* and *Nursing Service* will also be knowledgeable about advance directives and be available to provide appropriate counseling or answer questions. If the patient expresses a desire to formulate an advance directive to any member of the clinical staff, that individual should notify the treating physician. All activity related to the advance directive (e.g., education, counseling, execution) by any service must be documented in the progress notes.

f. If a patient is admitted to a special care unit at any time during a hospitalization, the *admitting nurse* in the special care unit should follow the procedure outlined in "part b" to ascertain if the patient has an advance directive or desires to formulate one. The inquiry set forth in 3b may only be conducted if it will not jeopardize or interfere with the treatment of the patient.

g. Any member of a clinical service may accept possession of a previously executed VA or non-VA advance directive at any time.

(1) The individual receiving the document will immediately present it to the *unit clerk* who will copy it, place the copy in the medical record, and label the outside of the chart. In addition, the individual receiving the document will notify the treating physician of its existence and will record this activity in the progress notes.

(2) The treating physician will review the document to determine its contents and, when appropriate, will discuss the document with the patient. District counsel may be called upon to assist in determining validity (see 2d(1).

(3) A social work service referral may be requested to provide any further education or counseling to the patient regarding the advance directive.

(4) In all cases, but especially if the previously executed advance directive is not valid according to VA policies, the patient will be encouraged to prepare a new VA advance directive.

h. Advance directives may also be executed in the outpatient clinic in accord with the policies and procedures outlined above.

i. Any oral statements made by the patient regarding advance directives or any

173

expression of wishes regarding life-sustaining treatment made to any health care provider at any time *must* be documented in the progress notes and the treating physician and unit or clinic clerk notified.

j. Advance directives must be reviewed periodically with the patient and/or surrogate decision maker by the treating physician and, where appropriate, the social work service to determine the directive's relevance to the patient's current medical and family status. Counseling and education will be provided to the patient. All reviews should be documented in the progress notes including the date of the review and name(s) of reviewers. The patient should place their initials and the date the review occurred next to their signature on the original and all copies of the advance directive document. Reviews will occur:

(1) At the patient's request;

(2) At each hospital admission;

(3) Whenever there is a significant change in the patient's medical condition;

(4) Whenever a patient is admitted to a special care unit (see 3f);

(5) At least annually for patients who remain hospitalized for prolonged stays.

k. An advance directive may be revoked at any time by the patient.

(1) This may be accomplished by destruction of the document by the patient or by some other person acting at the patient's request and in the patient's presence, by a signed and dated written statement by the patient, or by an oral statement by the patient.

(2) If a patient expresses a desire to revoke the advance directive, the time, date, and nature of the request should be documented in the progress notes by the treating physician or his or her clinical designee.

(3) The treating physician or his or her designee will write "REVOKED" in bold red print across each page of the advance directive. The "Advance Directive Inside" label should be removed from the chart until such time as a new advance directive is executed.

(4) The *social worker* will make an effort to locate each copy of the advance directive in the patient's or surrogate's possession and destroy such documents or label them "REVOKED." A note of this activity and which copies were destroyed or labeled should be made in the progress notes.

l. A patient may change his or her advance directive at any time.

(1) If a patient expresses a desire to change or modify his or her advance directive, the time, date, and nature of request should be documented in the progress notes by the treating physician or his or her clinical designee. The treating physician or his or her designee will write "CHANGED" in bold red print across each page of the advance directive.

(2) The patient will be encouraged to execute a new document. However,

the oral change may constitute an advance directive even if a new document is not executed.

   (3) The *social worker* will make an effort to locate each copy of the advance directive in the patient's or surrogate's possession and likewise label them "CHANGED." A note of this activity and which copies were labeled should be made in the progress notes.

m. The treating physician will have the authority to approve implementation of the advance directive.

   (1) To give approval, he or she must determine that:

      (a) the patient lacks decision-making capacity;

      (b) the treatment to be withheld or withdrawn is life-sustaining treatment;

      (c) the treatment to be withheld or withdrawn is treatment that the patient or his or her surrogate decision maker clearly directs to be withheld or withdrawn;

      (d) all administrative requirements have been fulfilled.

   (2) The treating physician will document in the progress notes along with written concurrence of a second VA physician (which includes residents) that the approval conditions listed have been met. Concurrence may be documented by counter signature on the progress note.

   (3) The treating physician will write an order indicating at a minimum, "Advance Directive To Be Implemented."

   (4) In cases involving a pregnant veteran, district counsel must be consulted prior to implementation (see paragraph 2d[1]).

n. When a surrogate decision maker is acting for the patient in making decisions regarding any medical treatments including life-sustaining treatments, the same determinations list in Section I, part 1, will be made by the treating physician, and a second VA physician must concur in writing.

   (1) The same informed consent standards will be applied to the surrogate decision maker as would be applied to the competent patient.

   (2) If no DPAHC or Living Will or Advance Directive has been executed and the patient lacks decision-making capacity and is not likely to regain it in a reasonable amount of time, either the court-appointed guardian of the patient or, if none, the patient's next of kin may represent the patient.

   (3) Some patients who lack decision-making capacity may not have a guardian, next to kin, or designated agent available or willing to act as a surrogate decision maker. District counsel may be consulted in these cases to initiate action to secure court appointment of a surrogate (see 2d[1]).

   (4) In cases where no surrogate decision maker has been designated, con-

sent to life-sustaining treatment will be implied until a surrogate decision maker is available.

(5) If the treating physician believes that the decision of the surrogate decision maker is not in the patient's best interest or does not reflect the patient's own desires, he or she may decline to implement the decision and the case will be referred to the Ethics Advisory Committee.

o. Any health care provider who does not want to participate in withholding or withdrawal of life-sustaining treatment for any reason will not be required to do so. In such cases, responsibility for the patient's care will be delegated to another health care provider.

p. Disputes among medical staff, or between health care staff and the patient or surrogate decision maker, may be referred to the chief of the service, chief of staff, district counsel, and/or Ethics Advisory Committee.

q. A decision to withhold or withdraw life-sustaining treatment never justifies providing less than humane care and total concern for the patient's welfare, comfort, and dignity. All members of the health care team will provide all forms of medically indicated treatment, which are not subject to the advance directive. Treating physicians are encouraged to write onto the order sheet those medical efforts that will be maintained to relieve suffering and to assure comfort and dignity.

4. **References:**

a. Department of Veterans Affairs, Veterans Health Administration Manual M-2, "Clinical Affairs," Part I, "General," Chapter 31, "Withholding and Withdrawal of Life-Sustaining Treatment."

b. Joint Commission for Accreditation of Healthcare Organizations, Accreditation Manual for Hospitals, 1992 Edition, "Patient Rights" chapter.

JOSE R. CORONADO, Director

VA Living Will/VA Advance Directive

To any medical facility in whose care I happen to be and to any individual who may become responsible for my health care:

If the time comes when I, _____ (print name), can no longer take part in the decisions affecting my health care and treatment, it is my intention while I am still of sound mind that this document shall stand as an expression of my wishes.

A terminal illness, for the purposes of this directive, is a debilitating condition that is medically incurable or not treatable in terms of available technology and can be expected to cause death. A terminal illness is also one in which death will occur whether or not life-sustaining treatment is used, and the application of life-sustaining treatment would serve only to artificially prolong the dying process. In addition, terminal illnesses shall include conditions where death is imminent, as well as debilitating conditions from which there is no reasonable hope for recovery (e.g., a coma or persistent vegetative state).

"Life-sustaining treatment" means medical care, procedures, or interventions, which when applied to a patient with a "terminal illness," would have little or no effect on the underlying disease, injury, or condition, and which would only serve to delay death. Such treatment may include, but is not limited to, resuscitation, artificial nutrition and hydration, mechanical ventilation, and dialysis.

If, at any time, I should have a terminal illness, as defined herein, as determined by my attending (or primary treating) physician, with the concurrence of another physician, I direct that such life-sustaining treatment, as defined herein, be withheld or withdrawn, and that I be permitted to die naturally with only the administration of such medical care and procedures deemed necessary to help make me comfortable.

In the absence of an ability to give directions regarding the use of such life-sustaining treatment, it is my intention that this declaration shall be honored as the final expression of my moral and legal right to refuse medical or surgical treatment and to accept the full consequences (including death) of such refusal.

I understand that this is a preprinted form. Therefore, any comments, restrictions, or additional instructions that I wish to make are described on the attached document entitled, "Treatment Preferences." The specific matters addressed in the attached document shall take priority over the provisions set forth in this document, if there is any conflict. THIS PARAGRAPH SHALL TAKE EFFECT ONLY IF MY INITIALS ARE ENTERED HERE: _____

I understand the full importance of this declaration and I am emotionally and mentally competent to make this declaration.

SIGNATURE _____ DATE _____

SOCIAL SECURITY NUMBER _____ DATE OF BIRTH _____ MOTHER'S MAIDEN NAME _____

We declare that _____ (print name) has signed this VA Living Will/ VA Advance Directive in our presence and that he or she appears to be of sound mind and free from duress at the time this instrument was signed. In addition, we declare that the signer of this document has affirmed that he or she is aware of the nature and potential consequences of this document and that it has been signed freely and voluntarily.

SIGNATURE OF WITNESS _____ ADDRESS OF WITNESS _____

SIGNATURE OF WITNESS _____ ADDRESS OF WITNESS _____

177

VA DPAHC (Durable Power of Attorney for Health Care)

I, _____ (print name) do hereby appoint

Name: _____

Address: _____

_____

Telephone: (work) _____ (home) _____

as my true and lawful personal care attorney in fact, my health care agent. This appointment shall take effect only if I am unable to make or communicate my own health care decisions. My health care agent shall be authorized to make any and all health care decisions for me except to the extent I provide otherwise in this or another document. My agent is specifically authorized to grant, refuse, or withdraw consent on my behalf for any health care service, treatment, or procedure. This authority expressly includes the withholding or withdrawal of life-sustaining treatments.

My health care agent shall have the authority to talk to health care providers, get information, and sign any forms necessary to carry out these decisions. I hereby consent to the release by VA, to my health care agent appointed hereunder, of any and all information from my medical records that is, or may be, relevant to enable or assist my health care agent to make decisions about my health care and treatment. This authorization to release information is intended to include any information related to drug abuse, alcoholism or alcohol abuse, infection with the human immunodeficiency virus, and sickle cell anemia.

My health care agent is instructed to follow the treatment preferences, if any, expressed by me in the attached document entitled, "Treatment Preferences," or similar document. If the other document does not assist my health care agent in making the decision at issue, I instruct my agent to follow those preferences that I previously expressed, when I was competent to make such decisions. If this information is not known or available, I trust my agent to make decisions that he or she believes to be in my best interests.

In the event the person I have appointed is unable, unwilling, or unavailable to act as my health care agent, I appoint the following as my alternate agent:

Name: _____

Address: _____

_____

Telephone: (work) _____ (home) _____

continued

VA DPAHC—cont'd

CHECK ONE:	❏ This document is to remain in effect indefinitely. ❏ This document is to expire on		INITIALS
ATTACHED IS A DOCUMENT CONTAINING ADDITIONAL INFORMATION TO GUIDE MY AGENT	❏ YES	❏ NO	INITIALS

SIGNATURE _____   DATE _____

SOCIAL SECURITY NUMBER _____   DATE OF BIRTH _____   MOTHER'S MAIDEN NAME _____

We declare that _____ (print name) appears to be of sound mind and free from duress at the time this instrument was signed. In addition, we declare that the signer of this document has affirmed that he or she is aware of the nature and potential consequences of this document and that it has been signed freely and voluntarily.

SIGNATURE OF WITNESS _____   ADDRESS OF WITNESS _____

SIGNATURE OF WITNESS _____   ADDRESS OF WITNESS _____

Treatment Preferences

I, _____ (print name) intend for this document to guide my health care provider and my health care agent, guardian, or representative and may be used in conjunction with a living will or durable power of attorney for health care document.

Below are listed some situations I may encounter. I recognize these cannot exactly predict what might happen, but I instruct my agent to use this information to the best of his or her ability in making treatment decisions for me and on my behalf.

A. TERMINAL ILLNESS WITHOUT EXPECTATION OF RECOVERY AND PERMANENTLY LACKING DECISION-MAKING CAPABILITY

If the situation should arise in which I am in a terminal condition, am permanently lacking of decision-making capability, and there is no reasonable expectation of my recovery, I direct that I be allowed to die a natural death and that my life not be prolonged by extraordinary measures. I do, however, ask that medication be given to me as necessary, to relieve pain and suffering, even though this may shorten my remaining life.
YES _____ NO _____ INITIALS _____.

B. PERMANENT UNCONSCIOUSNESS

Whether or not I am terminally ill, if I become permanently unconscious, I direct that life support be discontinued. YES _____ NO _____ INITIALS _____.

C. BRAIN DAMAGE—UNABLE TO COMMUNICATE

Whether I am terminally ill or not, if I become unconscious and have very little chance of

179

continued

Treatment Preferences—cont'd

ever recovering consciousness, and would almost certainly be very brain damaged if I did recover consciousness, I direct that life support be discontinued.
YES _____ NO _____ INITIALS _____

D. DOES LIFE SUPPORT INCLUDE FOOD AND FLUIDS?

The previous situations (A, B, or C) may occur such that life can be prolonged when food and fluids are provided by tubes or other invasive measures. These include TUBES IN THE NOSE OR STOMACH and INTRAVENOUS FEEDINGS. If one of the above situations develops, I direct that tubes or other invasive measures for providing food and fluids not be started. If they are started, they are to be discontinued in the following situations (see previous descriptions):

   A. Terminal illness   YES _____ NO _____ INITIALS _____

   B. Permanent unconsciousness   YES _____ NO _____ INITIALS _____

   C. Brain damage   YES _____ NO _____ INITIALS _____

I direct that although other forms of life-sustaining therapies may be withheld or withdrawn as directed by my agent, food and fluids are to be given or maintained.
INITIALS _____

E. TRIAL OF THERAPY

If am not terminally ill but recovery is very unlikely (5% or less chance of getting better), I request that trial of therapy be given as determined by my agent and my physician(s). This therapy may include (but is not limited to) mechanical ventilation, antibiotics, and artificially provided feedings. YES _____ NO _____ INITIALS _____

KEEP THIS DOCUMENT FILED ON TOP

Withholding/Withdrawal of Life-Sustaining Treatment

■ Do you possess a living will and durable Power of Attorney?
❑ YES   ❑ NO

■ If the answer is yes, could you furnish this hospital a copy of your signed document?
❑ YES   ❑ NO

■ Are you interested in further information on these subjects?
❑ YES   ❑ NO

Information brochure provided   ❑ YES   ❑ NO

_____   _____
(Signature)   (Date)

_____   _____
(Signature)   (Date)

REMARKS:

_____

_____

_____

_____

_____

_____

KEEP THIS DOCUMENT FILED ON TOP

Appendix B: VALUES HISTORY FORM

NAME: _____

DATE: _____

If someone assisted you in completing this form please fill in his or her name, address, and relationship to you.

Name: _____

Address: _____

_____

Relationship: _____

It is important that your medical treatment be **your choice.**

The purpose of this form is to assist you in thinking about and writing down what is important to you about your health. If you should at some time become unable to make health care decisions, this form may help others make a decision for you in accordance with your values.

The first section of this form provides an opportunity for you to discuss your values, wishes, and preferences in a number of different areas such as your personal relationships, your overall attitude toward life, and your thoughts about illness.

The second section of this form provides a space for indicating whether you have completed an Advance Directive (e.g., a Living Will, Durable Power of Attorney for Health Care Decisions, or Advance Directive for Health Care) and where these documents may be found.

Overall Attitude Toward Life and Death

What would you like to say to someone reading this document about your overall attitude toward life?

What goals do you have for the future?

How satisfied are you with what you have achieved in your life?

What, for you, makes life worth living?

What do you fear most? What frightens or upsets you?

What activities do you enjoy (e.g., hobbies, watching TV, etc.)?

How would you describe your current state of health?

If you currently have any health problems or disabilities, how do they affect: you? your family? your work? your ability to function?

If you have health problems or disabilities, how do you feel about them? What would you like others (family, friends, doctors) to know about this?

Do you have difficulties in getting through the day with activities such as: eating? preparing food? sleeping? dressing and bathing? etc.

What would you like to say to someone reading this document about your general health?

Personal Relationships

What role do family and friends play in your life?

How do you expect friends, family, and others to support your decisions regarding medical treatment you may need now or in the future?

Have you made any arrangements for family or friends to make medical treatment decisions on your behalf? If so, who has agreed to make decisions for you and in what circumstances?

What general comments would you like to make about the personal relationships in your life?

Thoughts About Independence and Self-Sufficiency

How does independence or dependence affect your life?

If you were to experience decreased physical and mental abilities, how would that affect your attitude toward independence and self-sufficiency?

If your current physical or mental health gets worse, how would you feel?

Living Environment

Have you lived alone or with others over the last 10 years?

How comfortable have you been in your surroundings? How might illness, disability, or age affect this?

What general comments would you like to make about your surroundings?

Religious Background and Beliefs

What is your spiritual/religious background?

How do your beliefs affect your feelings toward serious, chronic, or terminal illness?

How does your faith community, church, or synagogue support you?

What general comments would you like to make about your beliefs?

Relationships with Doctors and Other Health Caregivers

How do you relate to your doctors? Please comment on: trust; decision making; time for satisfactory communications; respectful treatment.

How do you feel about other caregivers, including nurses, therapists, chaplains, social workers, etc.?

What else would you like to say doctors and other caregivers?

Thoughts About Illness, Dying, and Death

What general comments would you like to make about illness, dying, and death?

What will be important to you when you are dying (e.g., physical comfort, no pain, family members present, etc.)?

Where would you prefer to die?

How do you feel about the use of life-sustaining measures if you were: suffering from an irreversible chronic illness (e.g., Alzheimer's disease)? terminally ill? in a permanent coma?

What general comments would you like to make about medical treatment?

Finances

What general comments would you like to make about your finances and the cost of health care?

What are your feelings about having enough money to provide for your care?

Funeral Plans

What general comments would you like to make about your funeral and burial or cremation?

Have you made your funeral arrangements? If so, with whom?

Optional Questions

How would you like your obituary (announcement of your death) to read?

Write yourself a brief eulogy (a statement about yourself to be read at your funeral).

What would you like to say to someone reading this Values History Form?

Legal Documents

What legal documents about health care decisions have you signed?

Living Will? _____ Yes _____ No
If yes, where can it be found? Name, address, and phone number.

Durable Power of Attorney for Health Care Decisions? _____ Yes _____ No
If yes, where can it be found? Name, address, and phone number.

Advance Directive for Health Care? _____ Yes _____ No
If yes, where can it be found? Name, address, and phone number.

Other? _____ Yes _____ No
If yes, where can it be found? Name, address, and phone number.

Values History Form: Suggestions for Use

Here is the **Values History Form** developed at the Institute of Public Law, University of New Mexico School of Law. The form **is not a legal document,** although it may be used to supplement a Living Will, a Durable Power of Attorney for Health Care, or an Advance Directive for Health Care, if you have these. Also, the Values History Form **is not copyrighted,** and you are encouraged to make additional copies for friends and relatives to use.

Why A Values History Form?

The Values History Form recognizes that medical decisions we make for ourselves are based on the beliefs, preferences, and values that matter most to us: How do we feel about independence and control? About pain, illness, dying, and death? What in life gives us pleasure? Sorrow? A discussion of these and other values can provide important information for those who might, in the future, have to make medical decisions for us when we are no longer able to do so.

Further, a discussion of the questions asked on the Values History Form can provide a solid basis for families, friends, physicians, and others when making medical decisions. By talking about these issues ahead of time, family disagreements may be minimized. And when decisions do need to be made, the burden of responsibility may be lessened because others feel confident of your wishes.

How Do I Fill Out the Values History Form?

The Values History Form asks a number of questions about issues such as: your attitude toward your health; your feelings about your health care providers; your thoughts about independence and control; personal relationships; your overall attitude toward life; your attitude toward illness, dying, and death; your religious background and beliefs; your living environment; your attitude toward finances; your wishes concerning your funeral. Simply answer the questions. The form also allows you to record both written and oral instructions you might already have prepared.

There are a number of ways in which you might begin to answer these questions. Perhaps you would like to write out some of your own thoughts before you talk with anyone else. Or you might ask family and friends to come together and talk about your—and their—responses to the questions.

Often simply making copies of the Values History Form available to others is enough to get people talking about a subject that, for many of us, is difficult and painful to consider. The most important thing to remember is that **it is easier to talk about these issues BEFORE a medical crisis occurs.** Feel free to add questions and comments of your own to those already provided.

What Should I Do With My Completed Values History Form?

Make certain that all those who might be involved in future medical decisions made on your behalf are aware of your wishes: family, friends, physicians, and other health care providers, your lawyer, your Pastor. If appropriate, provide written copies to these people. But remember that each of us continues to grow and change, and so the Values History Form should be discussed and updated fairly regularly, as preferences and values evolve. Consider attaching a copy of it to your Living Will, Durable Power of Attorney, or Advance Directive for Health Care, if you have one, or filing the Values History Form with your important medical papers.

Who Should Consider Preparing A Values History Form?

Everyone. While it has been customary to focus on older people, it is just as important that younger people discuss these issues and make their wishes known. Often some of the most difficult medical decisions must be made on behalf of these younger patients. If they had talked with families and friends, these decision makers could feel reassured they were following the patient's wishes.

What If I Do Not Have A Living Will or Durable Power of Attorney for Health Care?

Whether you sign either of these is entirely up to you, and laws governing these vary from state to state. For information and assistance, the following agencies might be of help:

Concern for Dying/Society for the Right to Die
250 West 57 Street, New York, NY 10107 (212) 246-6973

This agency will provide legal information about Living Wills and Durable Powers of Attorney for Health Care, as applicable in your own state. Please write to them at the above address. Because of the recent large volume of requests, expect a 4- to 6-week turnaround time. If you have an emergency, you may telephone them, but they caution that it is very difficult to get through on the telephone.

American Association of Retired Persons
For a single, free copy of the *Health Care Power of Attorney* booklet, please send a postcard with your name and address to: AARP Fulfillment (Stock No. D13895), 1909 K Street, N.W., Washington, D.C. 20049.

You might also contact your local Office of Senior Affairs, your State or Area Agency on Aging, agencies providing Legal Services for the Elderly, or your personal attorney.

We hope this Values History Form is of help to you, your families, and friends. Many people have commented that it is important to reflect not so much on "How I want to die," but rather on "How I want to LIVE until I die."

Appendix C: Code of Ethics and Guide for Professional Conduct of the American Physical Therapy Association

Purpose

This *Guide for Professional Conduct* (Guide) is intended to serve physical therapists who are members of the American Physical Therapy Association (Association) in interpreting the *Code of Ethics* (Code) and matters of professional conduct. The Guide provides guidelines by which physical therapists may determine the propriety of their conduct. The Code and the Guide apply to all physical therapists who are Association members. These guidelines are subject to changes as the dynamics of the profession change and as new patterns of health care delivery are developed and accepted by the professional community and the public. This Guide is subject to monitoring and timely revision by the Judicial Committee of the Association.

Interpreting Ethical Principles

The interpretations expressed in this Guide are not to be considered all inclusive of situations that could evolve under a specific principle of the Code, but reflect the opinions, decisions, and advice of the Judicial Committee. Although the statements of ethical principles apply universally, specific circumstances determine their appropriate application. Input related to current interpretations or to situations requiring interpretation is encouraged from Association members.

PRINCIPLE 1
Physical therapists respect the rights and dignity of all individuals.

1.1 Attitudes of Physical Therapists
    A. Physical therapists shall recognize that each individual is different from all other individuals and shall respect and be responsive to those differences.
    B. Physical therapists are to be guided at all times by concern for the physical, psychological, and socioeconomic welfare of those individuals entrusted to their care.
    C. Physical therapists shall not engage in conduct that constitutes harassment or abuse of, or discrimination against, colleagues, associates, or others.

1.2 Confidential Information
    A. Information relating to the physical therapist/patient relationship is confidential and may not be communicated to a third party not involved in that patient's care without the prior written consent of the patient, subject to applicable law.
    B. Information derived from component-sponsored peer review shall be held confidential by the reviewer unless written permission to release the information is obtained from the physical therapist who was reviewed.

C. Information derived from the working relationships of physical therapists shall be held confidential by all parties.

D. Information may be disclosed to appropriate authorities when it is necessary to protect the welfare of an individual or the community. Such disclosure shall be in accordance with applicable law.

1.3 Patient Relations

Physical therapists shall not engage in any sexual relationship or activity, whether consensual, or nonconsensual, with any patient while a physical therapist/patient relationship exists.

1.4 Informed Consent

Physical therapists shall obtain patient informed consent before treatment.

PRINCIPLE 2

Physical therapists comply with the laws and regulations governing the practice of physical therapy.

2.1 Professional Practice

Physical therapists shall provide consultation, evaluation, treatment, and preventive care, in accordance with the laws and regulations of the jurisdiction(s) in which they practice.

PRINCIPLE 3

Physical therapists accept responsibility for the exercise of sound judgment.

3.1 Acceptance of Responsibility

A. Upon accepting an individual for provision of physical therapy services, physical therapists shall assume the responsibility for evaluating that individual; planning, implementing, and supervising the therapeutic program; reevaluating and changing that program; and maintaining adequate records of the case, including progress reports.

B. When the individual's needs are beyond the scope of the physical therapist's expertise, or when additional services are indicated, the individual shall be so informed and assisted in identifying a qualified provider.

C. Regardless of practice setting, physical therapists shall maintain the ability to make independent judgments.

D. The physical therapist shall not provide physical therapy services to a patient while under the influence of a substance that impairs his or her ability to do so safely.

3.2 Delegation of Responsibility

A. Physical therapists shall not delegate to a less-qualified person any activity which requires the unique skill, knowledge, and judgment of the physical therapist.

B. The primary responsibility for physical therapy care rendered by supportive personnel rests with the supervising physical therapist. Adequate supervision requires, at a minimum, that a supervising physical therapist perform the following activities:

1. Designate or establish channels of written and oral communication.
2. Interpret available information concerning the individual under care.
3. Provide initial evaluation.
4. Develop plan of care, including short- and long-term goals.
5. Select and delegate appropriate tasks of plan of care.
6. Assess competence of supportive personnel to perform assigned tasks.
7. Direct and supervise supportive personnel in delegated tasks.
8. Identify and document precautions, special problems, contraindications, goals, anticipated progress, and plans for reevaluation.
9. Reevaluate, adjust plan of care when necessary, perform final evaluation, and establish follow-up plan.

3.3 Provision of Services

A. Physical therapists shall recognize the individual's freedom of choice in selection of physical therapy services.
B. Physical therapists' professional practices and their adherence to ethical principles of the Association shall take preference over business practices. Provision of services for personal financial gain rather than for the need of the individual receiving the services is unethical.
C. When physical therapists judge that an individual will no longer benefit from their services, they shall so inform the individual receiving the services. Physical therapists shall avoid overutilization of their services.
D. In the event of elective termination of a physical therapist/patient relationship by the physical therapist, the therapist should take steps to transfer the care of the patient, as appropriate, to another provider.

3.4 Referral Relationships

In a referral situation in which the referring practitioner prescribes a treatment program, alterations of that program or extension of physical therapy services beyond that program should be undertaken in consultation with the referring practitioner.

3.5 Practice Arrangements

A. Participation in a business, partnership, corporation, or other entity does not exempt the physical therapist, whether employer, partner, or stockholder, either individually or collectively, from the obligation of promoting and maintaining the ethical principles of the Association.
B. Physical therapists shall advise their employer(s) of any employer practice which causes a physical therapist to be in conflict with the ethical principles of the Association. Physical therapist employers shall attempt to rectify aspects of their employment which are in conflict with the ethical principles of the Association.

PRINCIPLE 4

Physical therapists maintain and promote high standards for physical therapy practice, education, and research.

4.1 Continued Education
  A. Physical therapists shall participate in educational activities which enhance their basic knowledge and provide new knowledge.
  B. Whenever physical therapists provide continuing education, they shall ensure that course content, objectives, and responsibilities of the instructional faculty are accurately reflected in the promotion of the course.

4.2 Review and Self Assessment
  A. Physical therapists shall provide for utilization review of their services.
  B. Physical therapists shall demonstrate their commitment to quality assurance by peer review and self assessment.

4.3 Research
  A. Physical therapists shall support research activities that contribute knowledge for improved patient care.
  B. Physical therapists engaged in research shall ensure:
    1. The consent of subjects.
    2. Confidentiality of the data on individual subjects and the personal identities of the subjects.
    3. The well-being of all subjects in compliance with facility regulations and laws of the jurisdiction in which the research is conducted.
    4. The absence of fraud and plagiarism.
    5. Full disclosure of support received.
    6. Appropriate acknowledgment of individuals making a contribution to the research.
    7. That animal subjects used in research are treated humanely and in compliance with facility regulations and laws of the jurisdiction in which the research experimentation is conducted.
  C. Physical therapists shall report to appropriate authorities any acts in the conduct or presentation of research that appear to be unethical or illegal.

4.4 Education
  A. Physical therapists shall support high-quality education in academic and clinical settings.
  B. Physical therapists functioning in the educational role are responsible to the students, the academic institutions, and the clinical settings for promoting ethical conduct in educational activities. Whenever possible, the educator shall ensure:
    1. The rights of students in the academic and clinical setting.
    2. Appropriate confidentiality of personal information.

3. Professional conduct toward the student during the academic and clinical educational processes.
4. Assignment to clinical settings prepared to give the student a learning experience.

C. Clinical educators are responsible for reporting to the academic program student conduct that appears to be unethical or illegal.

PRINCIPLE 5

Physical therapists seek remuneration for their services that is deserved and reasonable.

5.1 Fiscally Sound Remuneration
   A. Physical therapists shall never place their own financial interest above the welfare of individuals under their care.
   B. Fees for physical therapy services should be reasonable for the service performed, considering the setting in which it is provided, practice costs in the geographic area, judgment of other organizations, and other relevant factors.
   C. Physical therapists should attempt to ensure that providers, agencies, or other employers adopt physical therapy fee schedules that are reasonable and that encourage access to necessary services.

5.2 Business Practices/Fee Arrangements
   A. Physical therapists shall not:
      1. Directly or indirectly request, receive, or participate in the dividing, transferring, assigning, or rebating of an unearned fee.
      2. Profit by means of a credit or other valuable consideration, such as an unearned commission, discount, or gratuity in connection with furnishing of physical therapy services.
   B. Unless laws impose restrictions to the contrary, physical therapists who provide physical therapy services in a business entity may pool fees and moneys received. Physical therapists may divide or apportion these fees and moneys in accordance with the business agreement.
   C. Physical therapists may enter into agreements with organizations to provide physical therapy services if such agreements do not violate the ethical principles of the Association.

5.3 Endorsement of Equipment or Services
   A. Physical therapists shall not use influence upon individuals under their care or their families for utilization of equipment or services based upon the direct or indirect financial interest of the physical therapist in such equipment or services. Realizing that these individuals will normally rely on the physical therapists' advice, their best interest must always be maintained as well as their right of free choice relating to the use of any equipment or service. Although it cannot

be considered unethical for physical therapists to own or have a financial interest in equipment companies or services, they must act in accordance with law and make full disclosure of their interest whenever such companies or services become the source of equipment or services for individuals under their care.

B. Physical therapists may be remunerated for endorsement or advertisement of equipment or services to the lay public, physical therapists, or other health care professionals provided they disclose any financial interest in the production, sale, or distribution of said equipment or services.

C. In endorsing or advertising equipment or services, physical therapists shall use sound professional judgment and shall not give the appearance of Association endorsement.

5.4 Gifts and Other Considerations

A. Physical therapists shall not accept nor offer gifts or other considerations with obligatory conditions attached.

B. Physical therapists shall not accept nor offer gifts or other considerations that affect or give an objective appearance of affecting their professional judgment.

PRINCIPLE 6

Physical therapists provide accurate information to the consumer about the profession and about those services they provide.

6.1 Information About the Profession

Physical therapists shall endeavor to educate the public to an awareness of the physical therapy profession through such means as publication of articles and participations in seminars, lectures, and civic programs.

6.2 Information About Services

A. Information given to the public shall emphasize that individual problems cannot be treated without individualized evaluation and plans/programs of care.

B. Physical therapists may advertise their services to the public.

C. Physical therapists shall not use, or participate in the use of, any form of communication containing a false, plagiarized, fraudulent, misleading, deceptive, unfair, or sensational statement or claim.

D. A paid advertisement shall be identified as such unless it is apparent from the context that it is a paid advertisement.

PRINCIPLE 7

Physical therapists accept the responsibility to protect the public and the profession from unethical, incompetent, or illegal acts.

7.1 Consumer Protection

A. Physical therapists shall report any conduct that appears to be unethical, incompetent, or illegal.

193

B. Physical therapists may not participate in any arrangements in which patients are exploited due to the referring sources enhancing their personal incomes as a result of referring for, prescribing, or recommending physical therapy.

7.2 Disclosure

The physical therapist shall disclose to the patient if the referring practitioner derives compensation from the provision of physical therapy. The physical therapist shall ensure that the individual has freedom of choice in selecting a provider of physical therapy.

PRINCIPLE 8

Physical therapists participate in efforts to address the health needs of the public.

8.1 Pro Bono Service

Physical therapists should render pro bono publico (reduced or no fee) services to patients lacking the ability to pay for services, as each physical therapist's practice permits.

Issued by the Judicial Committee of the American Physical Therapy Association.
October 1981. Last Amended January 1996.

Code of Ethics of the American Physical Therapy Association

Preamble

This *Code of Ethics* sets forth ethical principles for the physical therapy profession. Members of this profession are responsible for maintaining and promoting ethical practice. This *Code of Ethics*, adopted by the American Physical Therapy Association, shall be binding on physical therapists who are members of the Association.

Principle 1: Physical therapists respect the rights and dignity of all individuals.

Principle 2: Physical therapists comply with the laws and regulations governing the practice of physical therapy.

Principle 3: Physical therapists accept responsibility for the exercise of sound judgment.

Principle 4: Physical therapists maintain and promote high standards for physical therapy practice, education, and research.

Principle 5: Physical therapists seek remuneration for their services that is deserved and reasonable.

Principle 6: Physical therapists provide accurate information to the consumer about the profession and about those services they provide.

Principle 7: Physical therapists accept the responsibility to protect the public and the profession from unethical, incompetent, or illegal acts.

Principle 8: Physical therapists participate in efforts to address the health needs of the public.

Adopted by the House of Delegates, June 1981. Amended June 1987 and June 1991

Appendix D: Standards of Ethical Conduct and Guide for Conduct of the Affiliate Member of the American Physical Therapy Association

Purpose

This *Guide for Conduct of the Affiliate Member* (Guide) is intended to serve physical therapist assistants who are affiliate members of the American Physical Therapy Association in the interpretation of the *Standards of Ethical Conduct for the Physical Therapist Assistant,* providing guidelines by which they may determine the propriety of their conduct. These guidelines are subject to change as new patterns of health care delivery are developed and accepted by the professional community and the public. This Guide is subject to monitoring and timely revision by the Judicial Committee of the Association.

Interpreting Standards

The interpretations expressed in this Guide are not to be considered all inclusive of situations that could evolve under a specific standard of the *Standards of Ethical Conduct for the Physical Therapist Assistant,* but reflect the opinions, decisions, and advice of the Judicial Committee. Although the statements of ethical principles apply universally, specific circumstances determine their appropriate application. Input related to current interpretations or to situations requiring interpretation is encouraged from Association members.

STANDARD 1
Physical therapist assistants provide services under the supervision of a physical therapist.

1.1 Supervisory Relationships

Physical therapist assistants shall work under the supervision and direction of a physical therapist who is properly credentialed in the jurisdiction in which the physical therapist assistant works.

1.2 Performance of Service

A. Physical therapist assistants may not initiate or alter a treatment program without prior evaluation by and approval of the supervising physical therapist.

B. Physical therapist assistants may modify a specific treatment procedure in accordance with changes in patient status.

C. Physical therapist assistants may not interpret data beyond the scope of their physical therapist assistant education.

D. Physical therapist assistants may respond to inquiries regarding patient status

195

to appropriate parties within the protocol established by a supervising physical therapist.

E. Physical therapist assistants shall refer inquiries regarding patient prognosis to a supervising physical therapist.

STANDARD 2

Physical therapist assistants respect the rights and dignity of all individuals.

2.1 Attitudes of Physical Therapist Assistants

A. Physical therapist assistants shall recognize that each individual is different from all other individuals and shall respect and be responsive to those differences.

B. Physical therapist assistants shall be guided at all times by concern for the dignity and welfare of those patients entrusted to their care.

C. Physical therapist assistants shall not engage in conduct that constitutes harassment or abuse of, or discrimination against, colleagues, associates, or others.

2.2 Request for Release of Information

Physical therapist assistants shall refer all requests for release of confidential information to the supervising physical therapist.

2.3 Protection of Privacy

Physical therapist assistants must treat as confidential all information relating to the personal conditions and affairs of the persons whom they serve.

2.4 Patient Relations

Physical therapist assistants shall not engage in any sexual relationship or activity, whether consensual or nonconsensual, with any patient while a physical therapist/patient relationship exists.

STANDARD 3

Physical therapist assistants maintain and promote high standards in the provision of services, giving the welfare of patients their highest regard.

3.1 Information About Services

A. Physical therapist assistants may provide consumers with information regarding provision of services within the protocol established by a supervising physical therapist.

B. Physical therapist assistants may not use, or participate in the use of, any form of communication containing a false, fraudulent, misleading, deceptive, unfair, or sensational statement or claim.

3.2 Organizational Employment

Physical therapist assistants shall advise their employer(s) of any employer practice that causes them to be in conflict with the *Standards of Ethical Conduct for the Physical Therapist Assistant.*

3.3 Endorsement of Equipment

Physical therapist assistants may not endorse equipment or exercise influence on patients or families to purchase or lease equipment except as directed by a physical therapist acting in accord with the stipulation in paragraph 5.3.A of the *Guide for Professional Conduct.*

3.4 Financial Considerations

Physical therapist assistants shall never place their own financial interest above the welfare of their patients.

3.5 Exploitation of Patients

Physical therapist assistants shall not participate in any arrangements in which patients are exploited. Such arrangements include situations in which referring sources enhance their personal incomes as a result of referring for, delegating, prescribing, or recommending physical therapy services.

STANDARD 4

Physical therapist assistants provide services within the limits of the law.

4.1 Supervisory Relationship

Physical therapist assistants shall comply with all aspects of law. Regardless of the content of any law, physical therapist assistants shall provide services only under the supervision and direction of a physical therapist who is properly credentialed in the jurisdiction in which the physical therapist assistant works.

4.2 Representatives

Physical therapist assistants shall not hold themselves out as physical therapists.

STANDARD 5

Physical therapist assistants make those judgments that are commensurate with their qualifications as physical therapist assistants.

5.1 Patient Treatment

Physical therapist assistants shall report all untoward patient responses to a supervising physical therapist.

5.2 Patient Safety

A. Physical therapist assistants may refuse to carry out treatment procedures that they believe to be not in the best interest of the patient.

B. The physical therapist assistant shall not provide physical therapy services to a patient while under the influence of a substance that impairs his or her ability to do so safely.

5.3 Qualifications

Physical therapist assistants may not carry out any procedure that they are not qualified to provide.

197

5.4 Discontinuance of Treatment Program

Physical therapist assistants shall discontinue immediately any treatment procedures which in their judgment appear to be harmful to the patient.

5.5 Continued Education

Physical therapist assistants shall continue participation in various types of educational activities which enhance their skills and knowledge and provide new skills and knowledge.

STANDARD 6

Physical therapist assistants accept the responsibility to protect the public and the profession from unethical, incompetent, or illegal acts.

6.1 Consumer Protection

Physical therapist assistants shall report any conduct which appears to be unethical or illegal.

Issued by the Judicial Committee of the American Physical Therapy
Association. October 1981. Last Amended January 1996.

American Physical Therapy Association

Standards of Ethical Conduct for the Physical Therapist Assistant

Preamble

Physical therapist assistants are responsible for maintaining and promoting high standards of conduct. These *Standards of Ethical Conduct for the Physical Therapist Assistant* shall be binding on physical therapist assistants who are affiliate members of the Association.

Standard 1: Physical therapist assistants provide services under the supervision of a physical therapist.

Standard 2: Physical therapist assistants respect the rights and dignity of all individuals.

Standard 3: Physical therapist assistants maintain and promote high standards in the provision of services, giving the welfare of patients their highest regard.

Standard 4: Physical therapist assistants provide services within the limits of the law.

Standard 5: Physical therapist assistants make those judgments that are commensurate with their qualifications as physical therapist assistants.

Standard 6: Physical therapist assistants accept the responsibility to protect the public and the profession from unethical, incompetent, or illegal acts.

Adopted by the House of Delegates, June 1982. Amended June 1991

Appendix E: Occupational Therapy Code of Ethics

The American Occupational Therapy Association's *Code of Ethics* is a public statement of the values and principles used in promoting and maintaining high standards of behavior in occupational therapy. The American Occupational Therapy Association and its members are committed to furthering people's ability to function within their total environment. To this end, occupational therapy personnel provide services for individuals in any stage of health and illness, to institutions, to other professionals and colleagues, to students, and to the general public.

The *Occupational Therapy Code of Ethics* is a set of principles that applies to occupational therapy personnel at all levels. The roles of practitioner (registered occupational therapist and certified occupational therapy assistant), educator, fieldwork educator, supervisor, administrator, consultant, fieldwork coordinator, faculty program director, researcher-scholar, entrepreneur, student, support staff member, and occupational therapy aide are assumed.

Any action that is in violation of the spirit and purpose of this Code shall be considered unethical. To ensure compliance with the Code, enforcement procedures are established and maintained by the Commission on Standards and Ethics. Acceptance of membership in the American Occupational Therapy Association commits members to adherence to the *Code of Ethics* and its enforcement procedures.

PRINCIPLE 1
Occupational therapy personnel shall demonstrate a concern for the well-being of the recipients of their services. (beneficence)

A. Occupational therapy personnel shall provide services in an equitable manner for all individuals.

B. Occupational therapy personnel shall maintain relationships that do not exploit the recipient of services sexually, physically, emotionally, financially, socially, or in any other manner. Occupational therapy personnel shall avoid those relationships or activities that interfere with professional judgment and objectivity.

C. Occupational therapy personnel shall take all reasonable precautions to avoid harm to the recipient of services or to his or her property.

D. Occupational therapy personnel shall strive to ensure that fees are fair, reasonable, and commensurate with the service performed and are set with due regard for the service recipient's ability to pay.

PRINCIPLE 2
Occupational therapy personnel shall respect the rights of the recipients of their services. (autonomy, privacy, confidentiality)

A. Occupational therapy personnel shall collaborate with service recipients or their surrogate(s) in determining goals and priorities throughout the intervention process.

B. Occupational therapy personnel shall fully inform the service recipients of the nature, risks, and potential outcomes of any interventions.

C. Occupational therapy personnel shall obtain informed consent from subjects involved in research activities indicating they have been fully advised of the potential risks and outcomes.

D. Occupational therapy personnel shall respect the individual's right to reduce professional services or involvement in research or educational activities.

E. Occupational therapy personnel shall protect the confidential nature of information gained from educational, practice, research, and investigational activities.

PRINCIPLE 3

Occupational therapy personnel shall achieve and continually maintain high standards of competence. (duties)

A. Occupational therapy personnel shall hold the appropriate national and state credentials for providing services.

B. Occupational therapy personnel shall use procedures that conform to the Standards of Practice of the American Occupational Therapy Association.

C. Occupational therapy personnel shall take responsibility for maintaining competence by participating in professional development and educational activities.

D. Occupational therapy personnel shall perform their duties on **the basis of accurate and current information.**

E. Occupational therapy practitioners shall protect service recipients by ensuring that duties assumed by or assigned to other occupational therapy personnel are commensurate with their qualifications and experience.

F. Occupational therapy practitioners shall provide appropriate supervision to individuals for whom the practitioners have supervisory responsibility.

G. Occupational therapists shall refer recipients to other service providers or consult with other service providers when additional knowledge and expertise are required.

PRINCIPLE 4

Occupational therapy personnel shall comply with laws and Association policies guiding the profession of occupational therapy. (justice)

A. Occupational therapy personnel shall understand and abide by applicable Association policies; local, state, and federal laws; and institutional rules.

B. Occupational therapy personnel shall inform employers, employees, and colleagues about those laws and Association policies that apply to the profession of occupational therapy.

C. Occupational therapy practitioners shall require those they supervise in occupational therapy related activities to adhere to the *Code of Ethics*.

D. Occupational therapy personnel shall accurately record and report all information related professional activities.

PRINCIPLE 5

Occupational therapy personnel shall provide accurate information about occupational therapy services. (veracity)

A. Occupational therapy personnel shall accurately represent their qualifications, education, experience, training, and competence.

B. Occupational therapy personnel shall disclose any affiliations that may pose a conflict of interest.

C. Occupational therapy personnel shall refrain from using or participating in the use of any form of communication that contains false, fraudulent, deceptive, or unfair statements or claims.

PRINCIPLE 6

Occupational therapy personnel shall treat colleagues and other professionals with fairness, discretion, and integrity. (fidelity, veracity)

A. Occupational therapy personnel shall safeguard confidential information about colleagues and staff members.

B. Occupational therapy personnel shall accurately represent the qualifications, views, contributions, and findings of colleagues.

C. Occupational therapy personnel shall report any breaches of the *Code of Ethics* to the appropriate authority.

Prepared by the Commission on Standards and Ethics (SEC)
(Ruth Hansen, PhD, OTR, FAOTA, Chairperson).
Approved by the Representative Assembly April 1977.
Revised 1979, 1988, 1994.
Adopted by the Representative Assembly July 1994.
This document replaces the 1988 Occupational Therapy Code of Ethics
(American Journal of Occupational Therapy, 42, 795-796),
which was rescinded by the 1994 Representative Assembly.

Appendix F: Canons of Ethical Conduct (American Board for Certification in Orthotics and Prosthetics, Inc. (ABC))

Foreword

The Purpose of the Canons of Ethical Conduct (Canons)

The profession of orthotics and prosthetics exists for the fundamental purpose of assisting patients in maintaining functional and productive lives. The public entrusts its confidence to those professional practitioners upon whose competence and sense of fairness and compassion they can rely. For the profession to thrive, the members must discharge their responsibilities in a fashion that will bring honor and integrity to that profession, thereby ensuring public confidence. The greatest effort possible should be made to satisfy each patient's orthotic and/or prosthetic needs. The relationship established and the manner in which the patient is served are essential factors for appropriate professional and ethical conduct.

Recognizing the significant role the orthotist or prosthetist plays in the physical and emotional welfare of the patient, the Canons were first drafted by the ABC in the late 1960s. Its purpose was to convey the philosophy and basic tenet that the welfare of the patient shall come first and to encourage and promote the highest standard of professionalism and ethical conduct. The original Canons have evolved to their present form consistent with this philosophy.

Committee on Character and Fitness

The ABC Board of Directors has tasked to the Committee on Character and Fitness the responsibility of maintaining the integrity of the ABC credential and the Canons of Ethical Conduct by reviewing complaints that allege violations of the Canons. The Committee shall review these complaints and make all decisions in accordance with the Rules and Procedures.

The Committee, which is comprised of three former ABC presidents, has accepted the responsibility of reviewing complaints in a timely and objective manner. Bound by confidentiality, the anonymity of the Committee is maintained to ensure a fair and impartial process, free from external influences.

Limited Authority of the Committee

Of course, the Canons cannot address every possible circumstance of unethical conduct. In fact, not all complaints are appropriate for Committee review. It is a practical impossibility for the Committee to police the entire profession. For example, the Committee lacks both the resources and authority to investigate complaints that allege criminal misconduct, Medicare or Medicaid (insurance) fraud, theft, discrimination, copyright, trademark and patent infringement, threats, libel, and slander.

These types of disputes can be addressed by various appropriate federal and state government agencies or in civil or criminal courts. It is only after these types of complaints have been disposed of by the appropriate government agencies and/or the courts that the Committee may begin to consider possible ethical violations of the Canons.

The Canons shall identify, in part, those practice areas over which the Committee may exercise authority. The Committee shall be responsible only for reviewing and determining violations of the Canons. Its role is not intended to be expansive but rather to ensure that ethical and professional services are rendered.

Interpretation of the Canons

The Canons should not be interpreted only as a means to identify conduct that is contrary to the philosophy of the profession, but also as a continual means to educate the practitioner on his or her responsibility to maintain and adhere to established ethical standards. The Canons should be interpreted consistent with the evolving practical day-to-day realities of servicing clients.

Character and Fitness Rules and Procedures

Upon request, the official Rules and Procedures, which include specific instructions and time lines for processing complaints, as well as a form on which to outline the complaint will be provided.

Canons of Ethical Conduct
Committee On Character and Fitness
American Board for Certification in Orthotics and Prosthetics, Inc.

I. Preamble

1.1 Introduction

The practice of orthotics and prosthetics (the "Profession") is a recognized allied health profession. The orthotist or prosthetist assumes specific responsibilities to the physician or other licensed health care prescriber, the patient, the public, the associates, and the Profession, itself. These responsibilities must be discharged with honor and integrity to assure the maintenance of public confidence in the Profession.

The Profession exists for the primary purpose of assisting patients to maintain functional lives. The orthotist and prosthetist shall be responsible for making the greatest possible effort to satisfy the patient's orthotic or prosthetic requirements. The manner in which the patient is served is the essential factor relating to appropriate ethical professional conduct.

Members of the Profession are responsible for maintaining and promoting ethical practice. This Canons of Ethical Conduct ("Canons"), adopted by the American Board for Certification in Orthotics and Prosthetics, Inc., (ABC) shall be binding upon all who hold ABC credentials.

1.2 Ethics, Custom, and the Law

Unethical conduct may involve violations of customs and usages of the Profession, as well as actions that violate the law. Failure to conform to these Canons, including conduct that violates moral principles, customs and practices of the Profession or the law, shall be subject to disciplinary action and ultimate determination by the adjudicative authority as established in the Rules and Procedures Regarding Ethical, Character and Fitness Complaints ("Rules and Procedures"). Such disciplinary action depends upon the particular circumstances involved and how the conduct in question reflects upon the dignity and integrity of the Profession.

Depending upon the circumstances, disciplinary action may range from a warning, reprimand, temporary suspension, decertification, censorship, or referral for criminal prosecution or civil action. Although decertification is the maximum penalty that may be imposed by the ABC for a certified orthotist or certified prosthetist who violates these Canons, each orthotist or prosthetist has a civic and professional obligation to report to the appropriate governmental body any and all evidence that may come to his or her attention involving the alleged criminal conduct of any orthotist or prosthetist relating to the practice of orthotics or prosthetics.

II. Practitioner Responsibilities to the Physician

2.1 Diagnosis and Prescription

The orthotist or prosthetist must receive a prescription from a physician or appropriately licensed health care provider before providing any orthosis or prosthesis to a patient. The prescription must state that the patient is ready for orthotic or prosthetic management. It is the sole responsibility of the physician or appropriately licensed health care provider, and not the orthotist or prosthetist, to determine the medical appropriateness of the orthosis or prosthesis.

2.2 Orthosis and Prosthesis Evaluation and Recommendation

It is the responsibility of the orthotist or prosthetist to recommend specific orthotic and/or prosthetic design. The orthotist or prosthetist shall recognize that each individual patient is different and deserves specific and responsive guidance from the orthotist and prosthetist. After evaluating a patient, the orthotist or prosthetist shall recommend to the physician or other prescribing health care provider, specific orthotic or prosthetic designs along with the reasoning for such recommendation. The orthotist or prosthetist shall be guided at all times by concern for the physical, emotional, social, and economic welfare of the patient. All decisions by the orthotist or prosthetist must be made with the understanding and intent that the patient's best interests are the primary concern.

2.3 Changes in Patient's Condition

When requested by the patient and/or the patient's physician or health care provider, the orthotist or prosthetist shall monitor and observe the patient's physical condition in connection with the orthotic and prosthetic care and the prescribed device to make certain the patient is responding appropriately. As soon as possible, the orthotist or prosthetist must notify the physician or referring health care practitioner and the patient of any change in the patient's condition related to the orthotic or prosthetic management plan and the patient's medical evaluation.

2.4 Provision of Services

The orthotist or prosthetist shall recognize the patient's freedom of choice in selection of the orthotic or prosthetic design and treatment. Professional affiliations, including employment and referral relationships, may not limit access to services and shall not affect the decision-making process of the orthotist or prosthetist. Orthotists' and prosthetists' professional practices and their adherence to the ethical principles of the ABC shall take preference over business relationships. Provision of services for personal financial gain of the orthotist or prosthetist, rather than for the need of the individual receiving the services, is unethical.

2.5 Altering Orthosis or Prosthesis

The orthotist or prosthetist may repair or adjust an orthosis or prosthesis without notifying the prescribing health care provider. However, such repairs or adjustments must conform to the original prescription. Any repairs, adjustments, modifications, and/or replacements that substantially alter the original prescription must be authorized by the physician or the prescribing health care provider.

III. Responsibilities to the Patient

3.1 Confidential Information

All information relating to a patient's background, condition, treatment, management plan, or any other information relating to the orthotist or prosthetist-patient relationship is and shall always remain confidential and may not be communicated to any third party not involved in the patient's care without the prior written consent of the patient or patient's legal guardian.

Patient information, which may be derived as a result of any orthotist's or prosthetist's peer review process, shall be held and always remain confidential by all participants unless written permission to release the information is obtained from the patient or patient's legal guardian. All patient information, which is derived in a workplace from a working relationship among orthotists and prosthetics relating to any patient, shall be held and always remain confidential by all parties. The confidentiality requirements set forth in this Section 3.1 shall be strictly adhered to by all certificants unless the information is required by court order or when it is necessary to disclose such information to protect the welfare of the patient and/or the community. In such event, all disclosures of confidential information shall be in accordance with applicable legal requirements.

3.2 Competency

All orthotists and prosthetists shall provide competent services and shall use all efforts to meet the patient's orthotic and prosthetic requirements. Upon accepting an individual for orthotic or prosthetic services, the orthotist or prosthetist shall assume the responsibility for evaluating that individual; planning, implementing, and supervising the patient; reevaluating and changing the program; and maintaining adequate records of the case, including progress reports.

3.3 Research

All orthotists or prosthetists shall support research activities that contribute to the understanding of improved patient care. In the event that any orthotist or prosthetist desires to engage in a research project or study, he or she shall first ensure that: (i) all patients affiliated with such projects or studies consent in writing to the use of the results of the study; (ii) the data and information regarding the patient remain confidential; (iii) the well being of the patient shall be the primary concern; (iv) the research is conducted in accordance with all federal and state law; (v) there is an absence of fraud; (vi) all data are fully disclosed; (vii) there is an appropriate acknowledgement of individuals making contribution to the research; and (viii) in the event that any acts in the conduct or presentation of research appear to be unethical or illegal, the orthotist or prosthetist shall immediately report the unethical or illegal conduct to the ABC and, if appropriate, the applicable law enforcement authority.

3.4 Trust and Honesty

All orthotists and prosthetists shall always be truthful and honest to the patient, physician, and public in general.

3.5 Fees and Compensation

Fees for orthotic and prosthetic services should be reasonable for the services performed, taking into consideration the setting in which the services are provided, the practice costs in the geographic area, the judgment of other related or similar organizations, and other relevant factors. The orthotist and prosthetist shall never place his or her own financial interest above the welfare of the patient. It is unethical for the orthotist or prosthetist to engage in false, misleading, or deceptive actions in relation to the ultimate cost of the services undertaken or furnished. Overutilization caused by continuing orthotic or prosthetic services beyond the point of possible benefit or by providing services more frequently than necessary is unethical.

Submission of false or misleading information in requesting reimbursement from third-party payers, including Medicare and private insurers, is unethical.

3.6 Practice Arrangement

Orthotists and prosthetists shall not: (i) directly or indirectly request, receive, or participate in dividing, transferring, assigning, or rebating any funds derived from a referral of a patient to any other individual or entity, whether affiliated with the orthotist or prosthetist or otherwise; or (ii) except for the fees earned for services performed for the patient, profit by means of a credit or other valuable consideration, such as an unearned commission, discount, or gratuity for providing orthotic and prosthetic services.

The orthotist and prosthetist shall refer all patients to the most cost beneficial service provider, taking into consideration the nature and extent of the problem, the treatment resources and availability of health care benefit coverage, and the likelihood of receiving appropriate and beneficial care. Participation in the business, partnership, corporation, or other entity does not exempt the orthotist or prosthetist, whether employer, partner, or stockholder, either individually or collectively, from the obligation of promoting and maintaining these Canons and the ethical principles of the ABC. If the orthotist or prosthetist is involved in an arrangement with a referring source in which the referring source derives income from the orthotist's or prosthetist's services, the orthotist or prosthetist must disclose to the patient that the referring practitioner derives income from the provision of the services. Orthotists and prosthetists shall advise their employer of any employer or employee practice that is in contradiction with these Canons and the ethical principles of the certification board.

3.7 Delay in Services

It is unethical for the orthotist or prosthetist to accept any prescription when the orthotist or prosthetist knows, or has good cause to believe, that the orthosis or prosthesis cannot be furnished within a reasonable period of time. In such instances, the orthotist or prosthetist must discuss the situation with the patient and prescribing health care practitioner.

207

3.8 Compliance with Laws and Regulations

Orthotists and prosthetists shall provide consultation, evaluation, treatment, and preventive care, in accordance with the laws and regulations of the jurisdictions in which they practice.

3.9 Consumer Protection

All orthotists and prosthetists shall report to the ABC any conduct that appears to be unethical, incompetent, or illegal. Failure to report any such behavior that is known to an orthotist or prosthetist shall be unethical.

3.10 Delegation of Responsibility

Orthotists and prosthetists shall not delegate any responsibility requiring unique skills, knowledge, or judgment to a less-than-qualified person. The primary responsibility for orthotic and prosthetic care performed by supporting personnel rests with the delegating orthotist and prosthetist. Adequate supervision is required to make certain that the patient receives the necessary and appropriate care.

3.11 Information to Patient

Orthotists and prosthetists shall endeavor to educate the public about the Profession through the publication of articles, as well as participation in seminars, lectures, and civic programs. All information provided to the public shall emphasize that each individual situation is unique and requires specific targeted evaluation and process. Orthotists and prosthetists shall not use, nor participate in any use of, any form of communication containing a false, fraudulent, misleading, deceptive, unfair or sensational statement, or claim. Orthotists and prosthetists shall not provide any consideration to any member of the press, radio or television, or other communication medium in exchange for professional publicity in a news item. All advertisements shall be identified as advertisements unless it is absolutely clear from the context that it is a paid advertisement.

3.12 Illegal Discrimination

The orthotist and prosthetist shall not decline to accept a patient on the basis of race, gender, color, religion, or national origin, or on any basis that would constitute illegal discrimination.

IV. Responsibilities to Colleagues and the Profession

4.1 Dignity and Status

208

All orthotists and prosthetists have the personal responsibility to conduct themselves in a manner that will assure the dignity and status of the Profession. Examples of unacceptable behavior include, but are not limited to, the misuse of the certification title; slander or libel of another; disparaging former employers; disparaging former employees; and misrepresentation of capacity as a provider of services.

4.2 Commercialization

The primary professional function of the orthotist and prosthetist is to develop the orthosis and prosthesis as part of a medical treatment team. However, the orthotist or prosthetist is not prohibited from providing related commercial services, such as furnishing soft durable medical supplies, as long as each patient and the public in general is made aware of the differences between the orthotist's and prosthetist's professional and commercial services.

4.3 Solicitation

It is unethical for an orthotist or prosthetist to either directly or indirectly solicit the patronage of individual patients by way of intimidation, threats, harassing conduct, undue influence, coercion, duress, unwarranted promises of benefits, or solicitation of a patient who is apparently in a mental condition that impairs his or her personal judgment to make decisions concerning the products or services being offered.

4.5 Education

All orthotists and prosthetists shall support quality educational programs and forums in academic and clinical settings. Each orthotist and prosthetist shall regularly attend appropriate seminars and lectures; review relevant periodicals, magazines and literature; and otherwise keep abreast of all developments in the Profession. It is unethical for the orthotist or prosthetist to participate in any programs, educational or otherwise, that falsely or deceptively represent the rights and privileges of the Profession.

V. Application of Canons to Registered Assistants, Technicians, and Accredited Facilities

5.1 Adherence to Canons

These Canons shall apply to all registered assistants, technicians, and accredited facilities who are credentialed by the ABC and who provide services that are related and incident to the orthotist and prosthetist.

5.2 Responsibility of Orthotists and Prosthetists

The orthotist and prosthetist, as well as the accredited facility supervising and/or employing the assistants and technicians, shall be responsible for their compliance with these Canons and shall use reasonable efforts to ensure that their assistants and technicians are in compliance with these Canons.

VI. Patient Care by Other Professionals

6.1 Concern About Care by Peers

The orthotist or prosthetist should exercise appropriate respect for other health care professionals. Concerns regarding patient care provided by other professionals should be addressed directly to that professional rather than to the patient. In the event that such concerns rise to the level of criminal violation, incompetency, malpractice, or violation of these Canons, the orthotist or prosthetist must immediately notify the ABC. The Committee will take appropriate action in accordance with these Canons and applicable law.

VII. Certification

7.1 Use of Certification

The certified orthotist and certified prosthetist shall use the fact that they are certified only as evidence of meeting the requisite standard of knowledge and competency in the profession as defined by the ABC. It is unethical for a noncertified orthotist or prosthetist to represent, directly or indirectly, that he or she is certified.

Appendix G: Statement of Ethics and Professional Conduct, American Association for Respiratory Care

In the conduct of their professional activities the Respiratory Care Practitioner shall be bound by the following ethical and professional principles. Respiratory Care Practitioners shall:

- Demonstrate behavior that reflects integrity, supports objectivity, and fosters trust in the profession and its professionals.

- Actively maintain and continually improve their professional competence, and represent it accurately.

- Perform only those procedures or functions in which they are individually competent and which are within the scope of accepted and responsible practice.

- Respect and protect the legal and personal rights of patients they treat, including the right to informed consent and refusal of treatment.

- Divulge no confidential information regarding any patient or family unless disclosure is required for responsible performance of duty or required by law.

- Provide care without discrimination on any basis, with respect for the rights and dignity of all individuals.

- Promote disease prevention and wellness.

- Refuse to participate in illegal or unethical acts, and refuse to conceal illegal, unethical, or incompetent acts of others.

- Follow sound scientific procedures and ethical principles in research.

- Comply with state or federal laws that govern and relate to their practice.

- Avoid any form of conduct that creates a conflict of interest, and follow the principles of ethical business behavior.

- Promote the positive evolution of the profession, and health care in general, through improvement of the access, efficacy, and cost of patient care.

- Refrain from indiscriminate and unnecessary use of resources, both economic and natural, in their practice.

Appendix H: Association of Rehabilitation Nurses Position Statement: Ethical Issues

The following position statement on ethical issues is the result of the efforts of an ethics issues task force established in 1991. Association of Rehabilitation Nurses members who have participated in the task force are Christina Berns, MSN RN CRRN CCRN; Beth Budny, MS RN CRRN CNA; Cheryl Graham-Eason, MS RN CRRN; Christina Mumma, PhD RN CRRN; Marion Phipps, MS RN CRRN FAAN; Patricia Quigley, PhD RN CRRN; and Terri Skipper, BSN RN CRRN. A board task force composed of Darlene Finocchiaro, MS RN CRRN, chair; Patsy Getz, MN RN CRRN; and Nancy Lewis, MSN RN CRRN; prepared the position statement, which was approved at the ARN Board of Directors meeting on September 15, 1994, in Lake Buena Vista, FL.

Ethical issues are of concern to all nurses. Rehabilitation nurses, in particular, encounter challenging ethical situations in the settings in which they practice. Nurses provide care to promote the health and well-being of individuals; this implies interactions between people, and it implies the seeking of what is good and of what leads to health and welfare. Ethics concerns the reasoned analysis and disciplined inquiry underlying a moral code, whereas morals are the conventions and norms of society—dictating what ought to be or should be done (Oermann, 1991). The tenets of *Code for Nurses with Interpretive Statements* (American Nurses Association, 1985) are the profession's moral code, and the interpretive statements explain, amplify, and analyze the ethical principles (Thompson and Thompson, 1981). Because it sets the parameters for the profession of nursing, *Code for Nurses with Interpretive Statements* governs the way in which rehabilitation nurses approach ethical decisions.

Ethical dilemmas are created when a choice must be made between difficult alternatives or when important principles conflict. Nurses practicing in the specialty of rehabilitation are confronted with numerous ethical dilemmas. Members of the Association of Rehabilitation Nurses have identified several ethical issues that are of concern to those practicing rehabilitation nursing; they appear below.

- Patients' rights, including the rights of adolescents (Adolescents are capable of understanding the decisions made in their name by their parents. If an adolescent was not involved in the decision-making process and does not agree with his or her parents' decision, the adolescent has no recourse regarding that decision. This leads to an ethical and legal conflict.)
- The use of restraints
- Do-not-resuscitate orders
- Advanced Directives, which imply nursing intervention and responsibility regarding living wills and durable power of attorney
- Management of clients who are disposed to self-destructive behaviors or suicidal gestures
- Issues related to health care reform and changes in how health care is performed and delivered including, but not limited to:
  - ❑ Access to health care
  - ❑ Cost containment

- ❑ Quality of health care
- ❑ Determining length of stay
- ❑ Providing care of the terminally ill clients and those with a shortened life span (i.e., those with developmental disabilities)
- ❑ Defining who meets the criteria for rehabilitation
- ❑ Dealing with clients' noncompliance with treatment and rehabilitation
- Confidentiality (which requires assessment of the value systems of both the patient and the nurse)
  - ❑ What information is given to the nurse by the client
  - ❑ What information can or cannot be given to the client by the nurse
- Substance abuse
- Abused clients
- The nurse-client relationship—when does it become too intimate, and when is intimacy between the nurse and the client appropriate?

Because ethical issues are of great concern for rehabilitation nurses, the Association of Rehabilitation Nurses developed this position statement.

Association of Rehabilitation Nurses Position Statement

The Association of Rehabilitation Nurses supports the 1985 American Nurses Association *Code for Nurses with Interpretive Statements* and the 1992 *A Patient's Bill of Rights* (published by the American Hospital Association) as important guides for ethical decision making. The Association of Rehabilitation Nurses makes the following additional statements:

1. The rehabilitation nurse acts as a client advocate.

2. The rehabilitation nurse recognizes the importance of clients' participation in the decision-making process and realizes that some clients do not and will not value independence and wellness as much as rehabilitation professionals do.

3. The rehabilitation nurse must always be concerned about the rehabilitation client's quality of life as defined by the client, which may be compromised by technological advances in health care. Advanced medical technology may prolong life but not improve the quality of life.

4. The rehabilitation nurse is responsible for providing information or assisting with the collection and interpretation of information that is necessary to resolve major ethical dilemmas.

5. The rehabilitation nurse stays informed of ethical issues that might affect rehabilitation clients and is aware of his or her own values and attitudes.

6. The rehabilitation nurse supports American Nurses Association's (1991) position statement on nursing and the Patient Self-Determination Act.

7. The rehabilitation nurse bases his or her decisions on the ethical principles of autonomy, beneficence, justice, and nonmaleficence.

8. The rehabilitation nurse participates in research and realizes that the benefits of research and human experimentation carry certain threats to human rights. To protect these rights when participating in research, the nurse considers the issues of informed consent, criteria for inclusion and retention of subjects, training of researchers, research dissemination, ethical supervision and accountability, and provisions for subjects' privacy and the confidentiality of results and findings.

Regarding the rights of patients, the Association of Rehabilitation Nurses holds the following beliefs:

1. All people have the right to receive rehabilitation services regardless of their age, race, gender, ethnicity, religion, or economic status.

2. All individuals have the right to receive full resuscitation, refuse appropriate treatment, request do-not-resuscitate orders, or request the discontinuation of life support.

3. All individuals have the right to expect that chemical restraint medication will be used only to modify or diminish maladaptive behavior that contributes to their distress and/or results in harm to themselves or others and with a defined plan of care, which includes a targeted outcome.

4. All individuals have the right to expect the appropriate use of the least restrictive physical restraints necessary to sustain body alignment, maintain personal safety, or protect themselves or others from injury. It is preferable to avoid the use of physical restraints altogether and consider nonrestrictive measures whenever possible.

5. All individuals have the right to expect that their care will include the use of proper medical rehabilitative resources, including placement in appropriate facilities, irrespective of any restrictive allocation of health care.

Glossary of Terms

Access—"The ability of an individual to receive a service that he or she needs or desires without being barred for reasons of social status, income, ability to pay, place of residence, or other factors that are not relevant to the adequate delivery of health care services" (Carroll-Johnson, 1993, p 44)

Advanced directives—A legal document written in advance of an incapacitating illness or injury in which people can provide for decision making about medical treatment if they are unable to make their own decisions (as specified in the Patient Self-Determination Act of the Omnibus Budget Reconciliation Act of 1990)

Advocacy—"An ethical process that requires health care providers to ensure that patients' rights are met" (Carroll-Johnson, 1993, p 44)

Autonomy—"The state in which individuals determine their own course of action according to a plan they choose; also known as *self-determination*" (Carroll-Johnson, 1993, p 44) (see **Ethical Principle**)

Beneficence—"A person's taking active positive steps to help others, prevent harm, and/or remove harm" (Carroll-Johnson, 1993, p 44) (see **Ethical Principle**)

Bioethics—"Ethics applied to health care; involves moral rules, principles, and values that guide relationships among health care professionals and their clients" (McCourt, 1993, p 44)

Confidentiality—"Handling of information in a way that contributes to patient's care and that does not disclose information to anyone who is not directly concerned with the patient's welfare" (Carroll-Johnson, 1993, p 44)

Durable power of attorney for health care—A legal document that an individual signs while competent to designate who will make his or her health care decisions if he or she becomes incompetent (e.g., comatose or confused) (Carroll-Johnson, 1993)

Equity—"The principle that cases that are the same should be treated alike and cases that are different should be treated differently. In health care, this principle is an attribute of a system that provides similar services to people who have similar health problems or needs" (Carroll-Johnson, 1993, p 44)

Ethical principle—"A statement containing a fundamental rationale in support of a state moral position or proposed action"; such principles include autonomy, beneficence, justice, and nonmaleficence (Carroll-Johnson, 1993, p 44)

Ethics—"The study of the nature and justification of general ethical principles that can be applied to special areas where moral problems are presented" (McCourt, 1993, p 230)

Justice—Giving others what is due or owed to them, what they fairly deserve, or what they can claim legitimately (Carroll-Johnson, 1993) (see **Ethical Principle**)

Morality—Traditions of belief about right and wrong human conduct (McCourt, 1993)

Nonmaleficence—"The duty of avoiding the intentional infliction of harm; not taking the risk of inflicting harm" (Carroll-Johnson, 1993, p 45) (see **Ethical Principle**)

Appendix H References

American Hospital Association: *A patient's bill of rights* (Management Advisory), Chicago, 1992, AHA.

American Nurses Association: *Code for nurses with interpretive statements*, Washington DC, 1985, ANA.

American Nurses Association: *American Nurses Association position statement on nursing and the Patient Self-Determination Act*, Kansas City, Mo, 1991, ANA.

Carroll-Johnson RM, editor: Glossary of terms, *Oncology Nursing Forum* 20(10)suppl:44-45, 1993.

McCourt AE, editor: *The specialty practice of rehabilitation nursing: a core curriculum*, ed 3, Skokie, Ill, 1993, Rehabilitation Nursing Foundation.

Oermann MH: *Professional nursing practice: a conceptual approach*, Philadelphia, 1991, JB Lippincott.

Thompson JB, Thompson HO: *Ethics in nursing*, New York, 1981, Macmillan Publishing.

Appendix I: American Nurses Association Code of Ethics

- The nurse provides services with respect for human dignity and the uniqueness of the client unrestricted by considerations of social or economic status, personal attributes, or the nature of health problems.

- The nurse safeguards the client's right to privacy by judiciously protecting information of a confidential nature.

- The nurse acts to safeguard the client and the public when health care and safety are affected by the incompetent, unethical, or illegal practice of any person.

- The nurse assumes responsibility and accountability for individual nursing judgments and actions.

- The nurse maintains competence in nursing.

- The nurse exercises informed judgment and uses individual competence and qualifications as criteria in seeking consultation, accepting responsibilities, and delegating nursing activities to others.

- The nurse participates in activities that contribute to the ongoing development of the profession's body of knowledge.

- The nurse participates in the profession's efforts to implement and improve standards of nursing.

- The nurse participates in the profession's efforts to establish and maintain conditions of employment conducive to high-quality nursing care.

- The nurse participates in the profession's efforts to protect the public from misinformation and misrepresentation and to maintain the integrity of nursing.

- The nurse collaborates with members of the health professions and other citizens in promoting community and national efforts to meet the health needs of the public.

Appendix J: American Speech-Language-Hearing Association Code of Ethics

Preamble

The preservation of the highest standards of integrity and ethical principles is vital to the responsible discharge of obligations in the professions of speech-language pathology and audiology. This *Code of Ethics* sets forth the fundamental principles and rules considered essential to this purpose.

Every individual who is (a) a member of the American Speech-Language-Hearing Association, whether certified or not, (b) a nonmember holding the Certificate of Clinical Competence from the Association, (c) an applicant for membership or certification, or (d) a Clinical Fellow seeking to fulfill standards for certification shall abide by this *Code of Ethics*.

Any action that violates the spirit and purpose of this Code shall be considered unethical. Failure to specify any particular responsibility or practice in this *Code of Ethics* shall not be construed as denial of the existence of such responsibilities or practices.

The fundamentals of ethical conduct are described by Principles of Ethics and by Rules of Ethics as they relate to responsibility to the persons served, to the public, and to the professions of speech-language pathology and audiology.

Principles of Ethics, aspirational and inspirational in nature, form the underlying moral basis for the *Code of Ethics*. Individuals shall observe these principles as affirmative obligations under all conditions of professional activity.

Rules of Ethics are specific statements of minimally acceptable professional conduct or of prohibitions and are applicable to all individuals.

Principle of Ethics I

Individuals shall honor their responsibility to hold paramount the welfare of persons they serve professionally.

Rules of Ethics

A. Individuals shall provide all services competently.

B. Individuals shall use every resource, including referral when appropriate, to ensure that high-quality service is provided.

C. Individuals shall not discriminate in the delivery of professional services on the basis of race or ethnicity, gender, age, religion, national origin, sexual orientation, or disability.

D. Individuals shall fully inform the persons they serve of the nature and possible effects of services rendered and products dispensed.

E. Individuals shall evaluate the effectiveness of services rendered and of products dispensed and shall provide services or dispense products only when benefit can reasonably be expected.

F. Individuals shall not guarantee the results of any treatment or procedure, directly or by implication; however, they may make a reasonable statement of prognosis.

G. Individuals shall not evaluate or treat speech, language, or hearing disorders solely by correspondence.

H. Individuals shall maintain adequate records of professional services rendered and products dispensed and shall allow access to these records when appropriately authorized.

I. Individuals shall not reveal, without authorization, any professional or personal information about the person served professionally, unless required by law to do so, or unless doing so is necessary to protect the welfare of the person or of the community.

J. Individuals shall not charge for services not rendered, nor shall they misrepresent,[1] in any fashion, services rendered or products dispensed.

K. Individuals shall use persons in research or as subjects of teaching demonstrations only with their informed consent.

L. Individuals whose professional services are adversely affected by substance abuse or other health-related conditions shall seek professional assistance and, where appropriate, withdraw from the affected areas of practice.

Principle of Ethics II

Individuals shall honor their responsibility to achieve and maintain the highest level of professional competence.

Rules of Ethics

A. Individuals shall engage in the provision of clinical services only when they hold the appropriate Certificate of Clinical Competence or when they are in the certification process and are supervised by an individual who holds the appropriate Certificate of Clinical Competence.

B. Individuals shall engage in only those aspects of the professions that are within the scope of their competence, considering their level of education, training, and experience.

C. Individuals shall continue their professional development throughout their careers.

D. Individuals shall delegate the provision of clinical services only to persons who are certified or to persons in the education or certification process who are appropriately supervised. The provision of support services may be delegated to persons who are neither certified nor in the certification process only when a certificate holder provides appropriate supervision.

---

[1]For purposes of this *Code of Ethics*, misrepresentation includes any untrue statements or statements that are likely to mislead. Misrepresentation also includes the failure to state any information that is material and that should, in fairness, be considered.

E. Individuals shall prohibit any of their professional staff from providing services that exceed the staff member's competence, considering the staff member's level of education, training, and experience.

F. Individuals shall ensure that all equipment used in the provision of services is in proper working order and is properly calibrated.

Principle of Ethics III

Individuals shall honor their responsibility to the public by promoting public understanding of the professions, by supporting the development of services designed to fulfill the unmet needs of the public, and by providing accurate information in all communications involving any aspect of the professions.

Rules of Ethics

A. Individuals shall not misrepresent their credentials, competence, education, training, or experience.

B. Individuals shall not participate in professional activities that constitute a conflict of interest.

C. Individuals shall not misrepresent diagnostic information, services rendered, or products dispensed or engage in any scheme or artifice to defraud in connection with obtaining payment or reimbursement for such services or products.

D. Individuals' statements to the public shall provide accurate information about the nature and management of communication disorders, about the professions, and about professional services.

E. Individuals' statements to the public—advertising, announcing, and marketing their professional services, reporting research results, and promoting products—shall adhere to prevailing professional standards and shall not contain misrepresentations.

Principle of Ethics IV

Individuals shall honor their responsibilities to the professions and their relationships with colleagues, students, and members of allied professions. Individuals shall uphold the dignity and autonomy of the professions, maintain harmonious interprofessional and intraprofessional relationships, and accept the professions' self-imposed standards.

Rules of Ethics

A. Individuals shall prohibit anyone under their supervision from engaging in any practice that violates the *Code of Ethics.*

B. Individuals shall not engage in dishonesty, fraud, deceit, misrepresentation, or any form of conduct that adversely reflects on the professions or on the individual's fitness to serve persons professionally.

C. Individuals shall assign credit only to those who have contributed to a publication, presentation, or product. Credit shall be assigned in proportion to the contribution and only with the contributor's consent.

D. Individuals' statements to colleagues about professional services, research results, and products shall adhere to prevailing professional standards and shall contain no misrepresentations.

E. Individuals shall not provide professional services without exercising independent professional judgment, regardless of referral source or prescription.

F. Individuals shall not discriminate in their relationships with colleagues, students, and members of allied professions on the basis of race or ethnicity, gender, age, religion, national origin, sexual orientation, or disability.

G. Individuals who have reason to believe that the *Code of Ethics* has been violated shall inform the Ethical Practice Board.

H. Individuals shall cooperate fully with the Ethical Practice Board in its investigation and adjudication of matters related to this *Code of Ethics*.

American Speech-Language-Hearing Association
Code of Ethics ASHA 36 (Mar, suppl 13), 1994, pp 1-2.

Index

A